Artifacts in Diagnostic Medical Ultrasound

Volume 1: Grayscale Artifacts

Martin Necas

For Melissa, Samuel, Madeleine and Benjamin, with love.

The National Library of New Zealand Cataloguing-in-Publication
Martin Necas
Artifacts in Diagnostic Ultrasound
Volume 1: Grayscale Artifacts
ISBN: 978-0-9872921-6-2 (paperback)

Published by High Frequency Publishing, Sydney, Australia 2017

http://ultrasoundbook.net

First published by Antegrade Ultrasound Solutions, Hamilton, New Zealand 2012

Also available in electronic version
ISBN: 978-0-9872921-7-9 (ebook)

Foreword

Ultrasound images are so prone to artifacts, it's little short of a miracle that we can see anything meaningful at all!

When the first sonographic images started to be produced in the 1960s, most doctors and scientists did not believe ultrasound would ever leave the experimental stage and become one of the leading imaging modalities. The notion that detailed and specific information about human anatomy and pathology could be gleaned from ultrasound echoes simply seemed absurd. Indeed, the first sets of published images were barely recognizable even to experts well versed in radiology and cross-sectional anatomy. The multitude of limitations associated with the behavior of sound in the human body, such as its catastrophic attenuation rates and its propensity towards artifact generation, posed enormous technological challenges to the developers of ultrasound devices.

Today, ultrasound is one of the most commonly used medical imaging modalities. Ultrasound images are not only highly meaningful, they can also be incredibly detailed with spatial resolution often greater than that of other flagship imaging modalities such as Computed Tomography or Magnetic Resonance Imaging.

To those who have made ultrasound imaging their profession, ultrasound images can also be incredibly beautiful. This is probably in large part because the operator is actively engaged in creating the image. Ultrasound is 80% science and 20% art. It's not a matter of pushing a button and obtaining an image.

Over the last four decades, manufacturers of ultrasound systems have gone to great lengths to improve image quality and reduce the generation and appearance of artifacts in ultrasound images.

And while fancy engineering tricks and complex hardware and software have helped reduce some artifacts, it is not possible to completely eliminate most artifacts because they are caused by the fundamental ways in which acoustic waves behave in soft tissue rather than being a product of limitations in equipment or signal processing. For this reason, ultrasound artifacts affect every ultrasound image and they are here to stay.

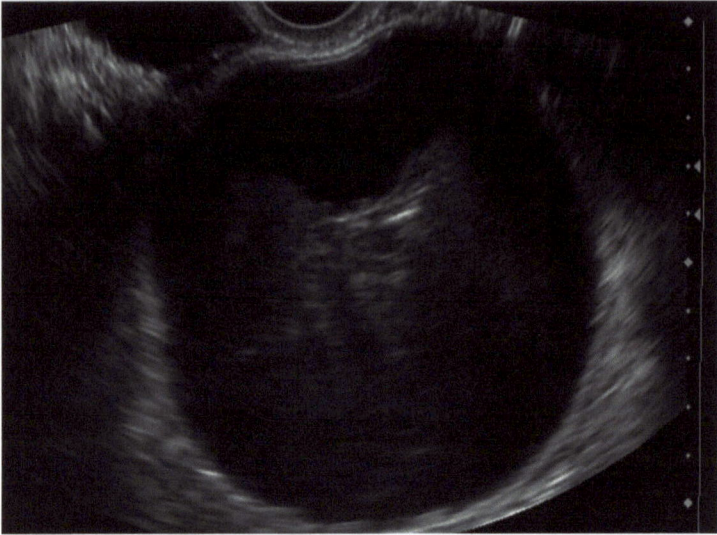

Figure 1: This image shows a benign simple ovarian cyst that was initially thought to represent a complex, predominantly solid ovarian mass. The solid internal contents are completely artifactual and are due to range ambiguity.

More often than not, artifacts are readily recognized by the operator and pose only a minor nuisance. But on occasion a cunning artifact will confuse even the most astute ultrasound practitioner.

The purpose of this book is to demystify artifacts, expose their true nature and offer you many tools to recognize, eliminate and circumvent even the most stubborn artifacts.

I hope you enjoy this book.

Martin Necas

Acknowledgements

I would like to acknowledge the many expert sonographers, scientists, radiologists and lecturers who have inspired me over the years to further my knowledge in ultrasound. I would like to thank Joan Baker who was instrumental in launching my career in sonography. Most of what I know about ultrasound physics I have learned from Roger Gent whose lectures I have attended on many occasions and whose textbook I have read from cover to cover multiple times.

I have fond memories of all the ultrasound departments where I have worked and acquired invaluable clinical experience including: Swedish Medical Centre in Seattle, Waikato Hospital in Hamilton and MIA Victoria in Melbourne, to name a few. I would also like to acknowledge my good friends and esteemed colleagues at the Australasian Society for Ultrasound in Medicine. It has been a pleasure and a privilege to work with so many outstanding ultrasound experts.

I am grateful for the advice, insightful comments and words of encouragement I have received in writing this book from Robert Gill, David Ferrar, Peter Stone, Stephen Bird, Mike Heath, Rex de Ryke, Wendy Barber, Karen Robertson and many other colleagues.

I would like to thank Dana McKay and Stephanie Chamberlin for their meticulous editorial review of the text and Tim Bromhead for his graphics design expertise. Finally and most importantly, I would like to thank my wife Melissa and children Samuel and Madeleine for their support, love and patience.

About this book

> You only recognize what you look for, and you only look for what you know.

Roger Gent

This book is written for medical professionals and students of ultrasound who are already using ultrasound technology in clinical practice. The book assumes basic background knowledge of acoustic principles, ultrasound technology and sufficient clinical background to interpret ultrasound images.

For more information on acoustics and ultrasound technology, readers are encouraged to refer to the many excellent texts in this field. In particular, the author recommends:

- Gill, RW 2012, The Physics and Technology of Diagnostic Ultrasound: A Practitioner's Guide, High Frequency Publishing, Sydney, https://www.ultrasoundbook.net.

- Gent, R 1996, Applied Physics and Technology of Diagnostic Ultrasound, out of print but available in PDF through the Australasian Society for Ultrasound in Medicine.

- Hedrick, WR, Hykes, DL & Starchman, DE 2004, Ultrasound Physics and Instrumentation, 4th ed (or later), Mosby.

- Kremkau, FW 2005, Diagnostic Ultrasound: Principles and Instruments, 7th ed (or later), Saunders.

About the author

Martin Necas works as a senior ultrasound practitioner and clinical instructor in Hamilton, New Zealand. Martin completed training in general and vascular ultrasound in Seattle, USA in 1996 and subsequently attained a Master's degree in Medical Sonography at the University of South Australia, Adelaide. Martin has practised diagnostic ultrasound in USA, New Zealand and Australia in a wide variety of clinical settings ranging from tertiary teaching hospitals to private specialist centers. Martin is an ultrasound enthusiast, clinical instructor, lecturer and a prolific conference speaker having presented over 100 conference presentations in the last 15 years.

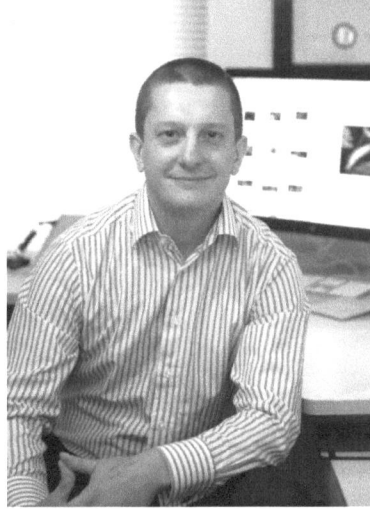

In this book, Martin draws on his extensive clinical and academic experience to deliver a detailed overview of ultrasound artifacts, their causation, clinical impacts and methods for reducing, eliminating and circumventing artifacts.

This book represents the largest collection of ultrasound artifacts images ever published in a single volume.

Contents

Chapter 1

Introduction to Artifacts

Ultrasound artifacts represent a wide range of misleading ultrasound appearances that do not accurately represent anatomical structures or physiologic events. In this chapter, we will discover various types of artifacts and the root causes of their existence.

1.1 What is an artifact?

An ultrasound system sends acoustic pulses into the patient and receives echoes that are generated by tissue reflectors.

In B-mode imaging, the depth of the reflector is calculated from the time taken between pulse generation and echo reception using the average speed of sound (1540m/s) in soft tissue as a constant. Echo strength (amplitude) is encoded as brightness.

In color, power and spectral Doppler, the returning echoes are further subjected to analysis for Doppler shifts.

In order for the ultrasound imaging system to analyze returning echoes and display them as images, a number of basic assumptions are made:

1   Ultrasound pulse travels in a straight line during transmission and echoes follow the same straight path.

2   Speed of sound in the body is a constant (1540m/s).

3   Attenuation rate is uniform and predictable.

4   Two comparable tissue reflectors in a similar location will generate a comparable echo amplitude.

5   The beam dimensions are small in height (axial), width (lateral) and thickness (slice thickness).

6   Echoes originate only from the central axis of the beam.

7   Each reflector only generates one echo.

8   The arriving echo was generated by the last emitted ultrasound pulse, not by any preceding pulses.

9   The rate of image acquisition exceeds the rate of physiologic events and the rate of transducer movement.

10 The operator is utilizing the system appropriately.

11 All system controls have been adjusted correctly.

12 The transducer elements and electronic system components are functioning normally and without interference from surrounding equipment.

Unfortunately sound (or in this case ultrasound) often fails to obey these convenient rules of pulse propagation, echo generation, signal reception and image processing.

Furthermore, the image acquisition rate may sometimes be too slow for rapid physiologic events, leading to a range of temporal display problems.

Finally, the operator (sonographer, sonologist) may sometimes play a significant role in creating circumstances for artifacts to occur. An example is shown in Figure 1.1.

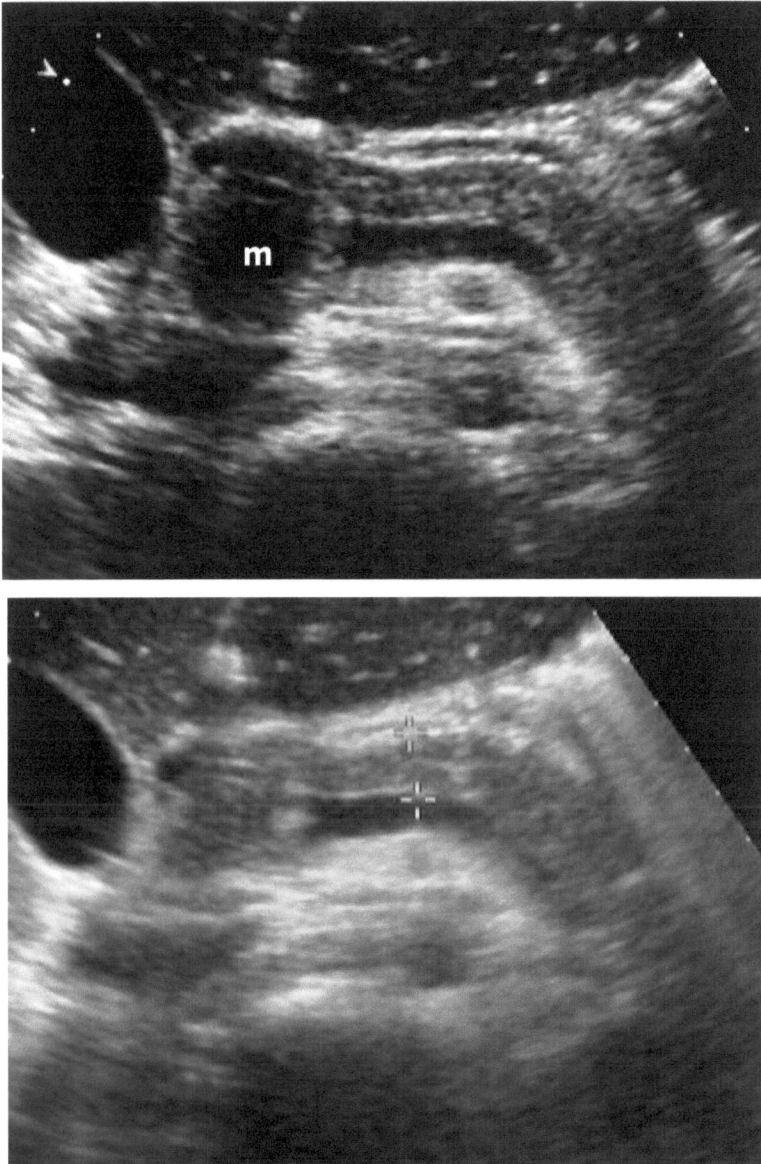

Figure 1.1: (Top) The sonographer used a non-uniform window (falciform ligament and ligamentum teres) to visualize the head of the pancreas. The appearance is highly worrying and suggests the presence of a pancreatic head mass (m). (Bottom) Review of the same area from a different angle revealed a normal pancreatic head.

1.2 General causes of artifacts

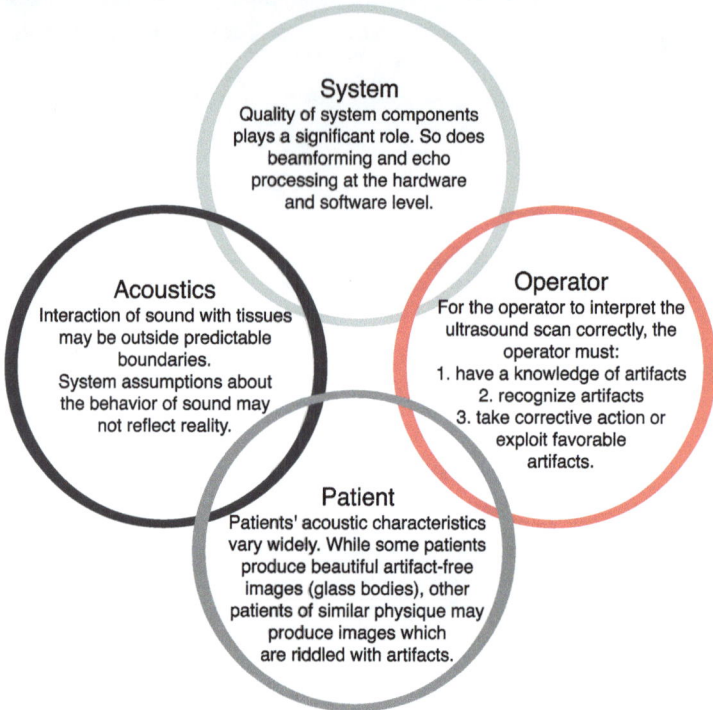

System
Quality of system components plays a significant role. So does beamforming and echo processing at the hardware and software level.

Acoustics
Interaction of sound with tissues may be outside predictable boundaries.
System assumptions about the behavior of sound may not reflect reality.

Operator
For the operator to interpret the ultrasound scan correctly, the operator must:
1. have a knowledge of artifacts
2. recognize artifacts
3. take corrective action or exploit favorable artifacts.

Patient
Patients' acoustic characteristics vary widely. While some patients produce beautiful artifact-free images (glass bodies), other patients of similar physique may produce images which are riddled with artifacts.

1.3 Sorting out the "truth"

While ultrasound artifacts do not accurately reflect reality, to the ultrasound system artifacts appear perfectly "real". Artifacts represent real echoes or the real absence of echoes, however, they do not represent real structures the way the operator would expect these to appear. Alternatively, the operator may misinterpret artifacts as real structures.

It is the operator's responsibility to determine whether the image accurately represents reality or not. It is useful to know:

1   what types of artifacts exist;
2   how each artifact arises;
3   the causative agent(s) for each type of artifact;

4   the system assumptions that have been violated;

5   the range of appearance of each artifact;

6   diagnostic uses of artifacts;

7   how to accentuate and use diagnostically useful artifacts;

8   how to reduce, eliminate or circumvent unhelpful or diagnostically detrimental artifacts.

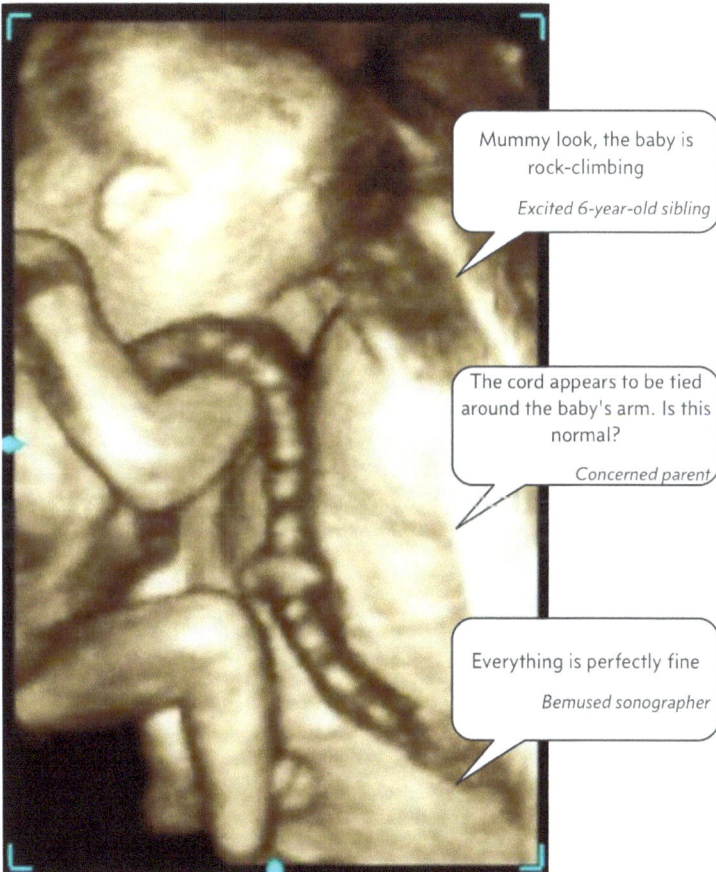

Figure 1.2: Determining what is real requires technical as well as clinical expertise.

1.4 Optical artifacts

> Reverberation is caused by bodies of a bright nature with a flat
> and semi opaque surface which, when the light strikes upon
> them, throw it back again, like the rebound of a ball, to the
> former object.

The Notebooks of Leonardo Da Vinci, 1452-1529

The above quote is a testament to Leonardo Da Vinci's astonishing insights into optical reverberation.

While light and sound behave quite differently, there are a number of parallels between ultrasound imaging and photography which may help explain many acoustic concepts. Some examples of optical artifacts are included on the following pages.

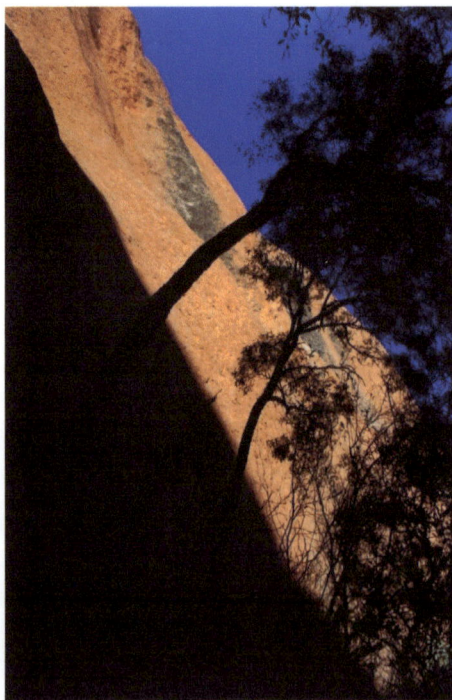

Figure 1.3: Shadowing can be observed both in optical and acoustic images.

Attenuation and scattering

This photograph was obtained in dense fog and the image of the building appears hazy. Light reflecting from the building is attenuated by the fog.

Another principle that can be seen in this image is that of scatter. Each particle of fog scatters light in multiple directions. In ultrasound imaging, the vast majority of soft tissue reflectors behave as scatterers.

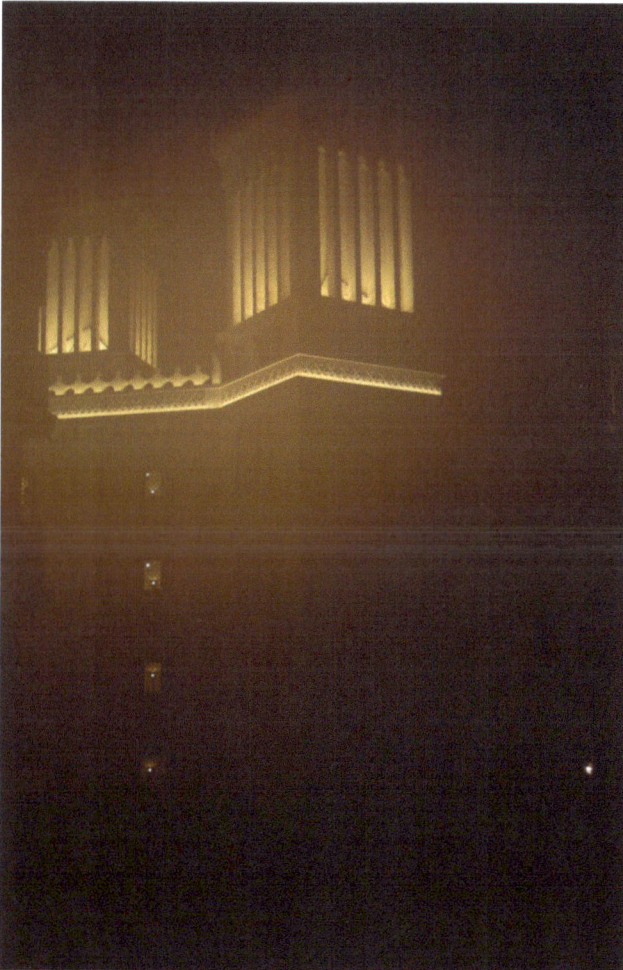

Figure 1.4: Dense fog scatters and attenuates light in a similar way to the scattering and attenuation of sound by soft tissues.

Curved mirror

Light reflects from a mirror at the same angle at which it strikes the mirror. The mirror's geometry therefore determines the way in which light will reflect and the appearance of the mirrored object. A straight mirror will preserve the size and proportionality of the reflected objects.

A concave mirror (see Figure 1.5) has a "slimming" effect. A convex mirror has the opposite (widening) effect. An irregular mirror (see Figure 1.6) will cause irregularity in the reflected image.

All of these scenarios can be encountered with acoustic mirrors as well. An entire chapter will be dedicated to mirror image artifacts.

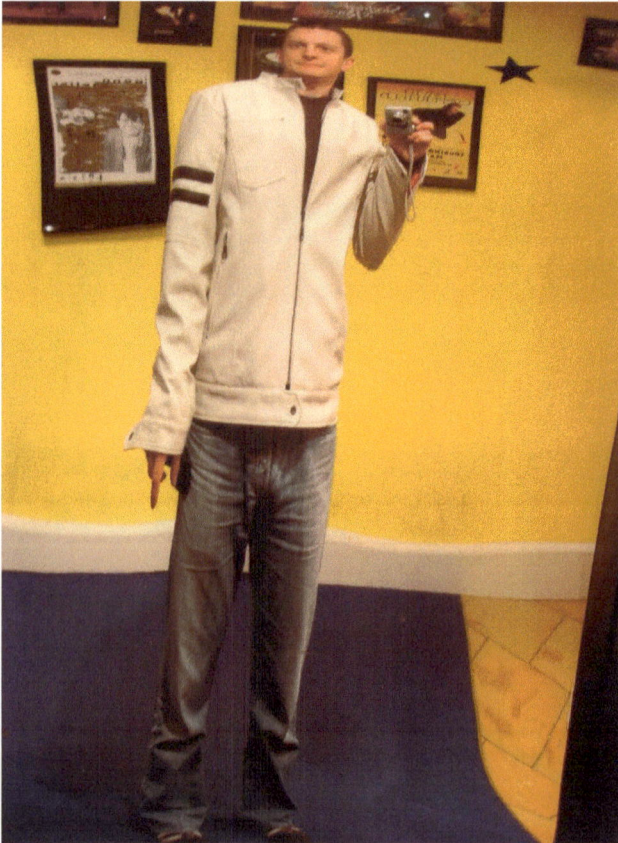

Figure 1.5: Distorted image of the author caused by a curved mirror.

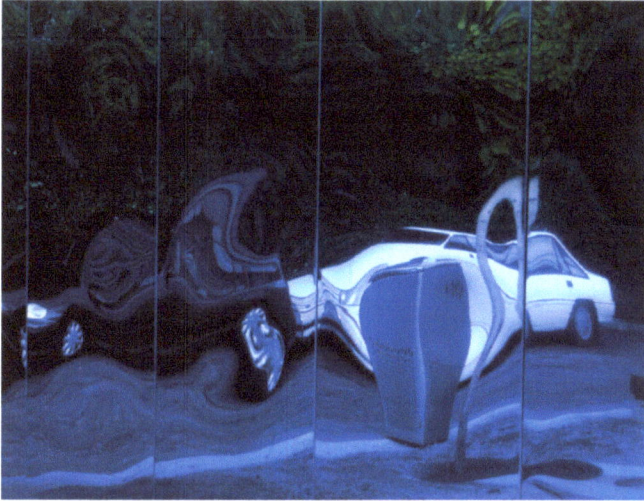

Figure 1.6: A more severely distorted image caused by an irregularly shaped mirror.

Partial mirror effect

A mirror may not cause complete reflection of light or sound.

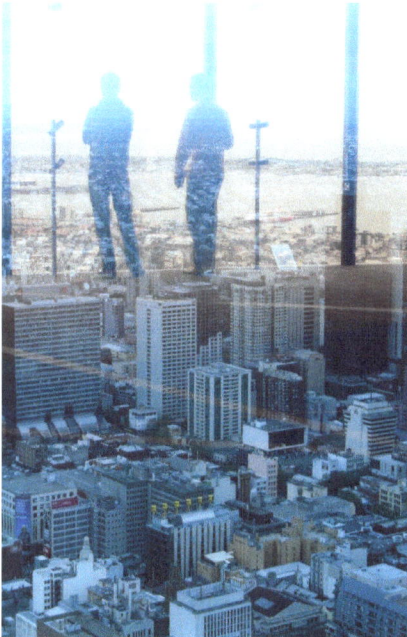

This photograph shows the glass pane of a high rise building acting as a partial mirror. The two figures seen "floating" above the city scape are reflections.

The partial mirror also allows light from the cityscape to get through.

Partial mirrors also occur in ultrasound imaging.

Refraction

Optical refraction is responsible for several well known effects. One is the apparent "bending" of a straight object submerged in a glass of water (see Figure 1.7).

A simple instrument for bending light and splitting it into its constituent wavelengths is a prism. Droplets of rain can also act in this way producing the beautiful optical effect of the rainbow.

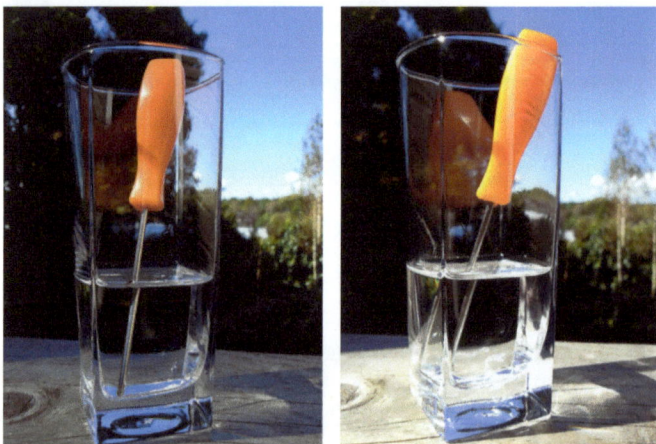

Figure 1.7: Distorted images caused by refraction.

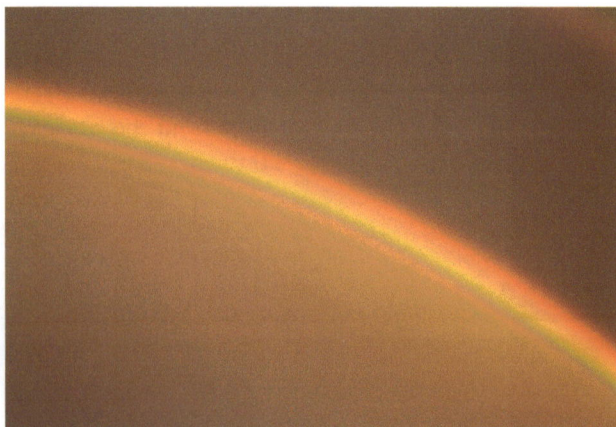

Figure 1.8: Rainbows are caused by refraction of sunlight.

Motion artifacts

Motion artifacts (also sometimes known as temporal localization artifacts) occur when the rate of the imaged event exceeds the rate of image acquisition. This leads to image smearing or may result in multiple separate events being captured in one image.

In ultrasound imaging, motion artifacts may happen for a number of reasons. For example, the imaged event (such as cardiac contraction) may be very fast. Alternatively, the system parameters and settings result in very slow frame rates (4D imaging). Patient movement and fast transducer movement may also result in motion artifacts.

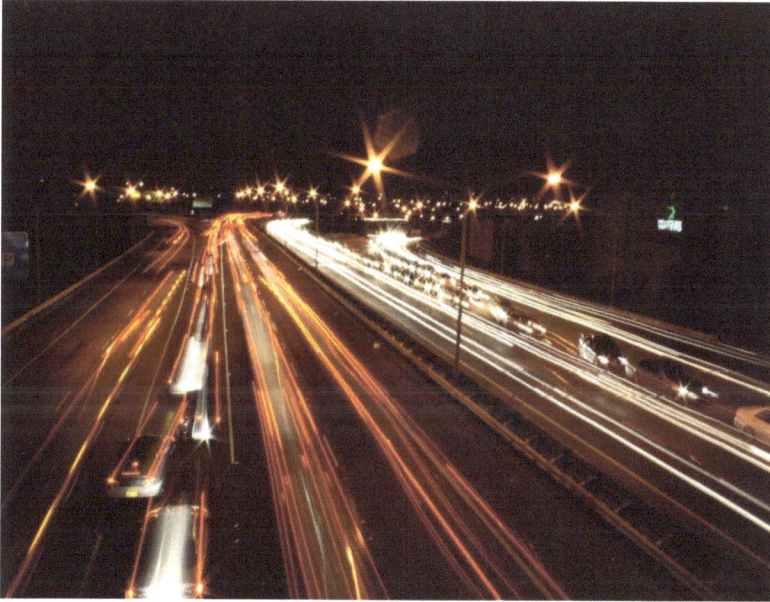

Figure 1.9: Traffic photograph showing dramatic motion artifact.

Chapter 2

Acoustic Speckle

Close inspection of ultrasound images reveals that anatomical structures are composed of discrete dots. This random distribution of echo amplitudes even within highly homogeneous tissues is known as acoustic speckle. Speckle is more of an acoustic fact than artifact.

Causative mechanisms

Acoustic speckle refers to the random variation in brightness of ultrasound reflectors, even within highly uniform homogeneous tissues. Speckle is the result of echo interference from a number of small scattering bodies within the ultrasound beam. The apparent location of bright speckle reflectors does not necessarily correspond to the location of a highly reflective interface.

The generation of speckle can be likened to throwing a handful of marbles into a pond. Each marble generates a circular propagating wave. These waves combine together through the effects of constructive or destructive interference. The location of the highest wave does not necessarily represent the location where a marble impacted the water. Similarly, the highest amplitude point within a region of speckle will not necessarily represent the true location of highly reflective interfaces.

Which system assumptions have been breached?

Two comparable tissue reflectors in a similar location will generate comparable echo amplitude.

Typical appearance

The typical appearance of speckle is in fact the normal appearance of an ultrasound image, where soft tissue structures appear composed of discrete dots.

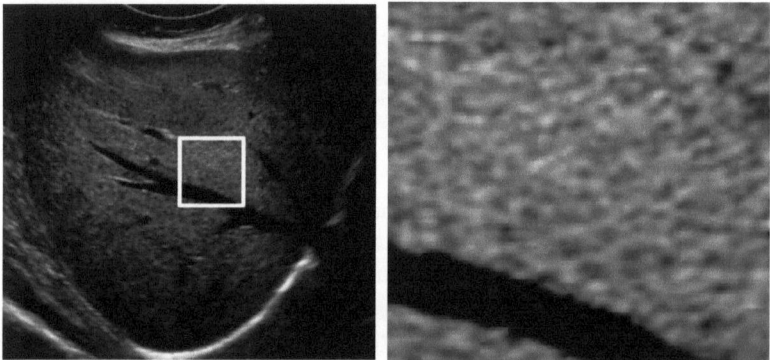

Figure 2.1: At first glance, this transverse image of the liver appears relatively smooth and uniform (left image). However, closer inspection of an enlarged segment of the image reveals the flecked nature of the echo distribution due to acoustic speckle (right image).

Can this artifact be reduced, eliminated or circumvented?

Three main speckle reduction technologies are available to sonographers:

1   The simplest (and historically earliest) attempt by manufacturers of ultrasound systems to reduce the appearance of acoustic speckle was the introduction of frame averaging also known as persistence. The use of high persistence tends to smooth images somewhat, but not very well. This is because acoustic speckle is highly angle dependent and imaging the same structure from the same angle tends to produce the identical speckle pattern. For persistence to be effective, a small amount of movement is required.

2   To reduce speckle, the structures within the field of view need to be interrogated at a variety of angles, each giving a different speckle pattern. Putting these images together like a series of transparencies results in a dramatic reduction in speckle. The technology that achieves this is known as spatial image compounding. Ultrasound manufacturers like to attach catchy terms to their proprietary form of spatial image compounding: SonoCT (Philips), SieClear (Siemens), ApliPure (Toshiba), Crossbeam (GE).

3   Ultrasound manufacturers also apply a range of mathematical algorithms to ultrasound images in an effort to smooth the image and reduce the appearance of speckle. On some systems the sonographer can adjust how much the function impacts the image, on others it may only be switched on or off. As with spatial compounding, proprietary mathematical algorithms carry various names, for example Xres (Philips) and SRI (Speckle Reduction Imaging on GE systems).

Is this artifact diagnostically useful?

Speckle is generally undesirable and large amounts of engineering effort have gone into the development of sophisticated hardware and software to counter the effects of speckle.

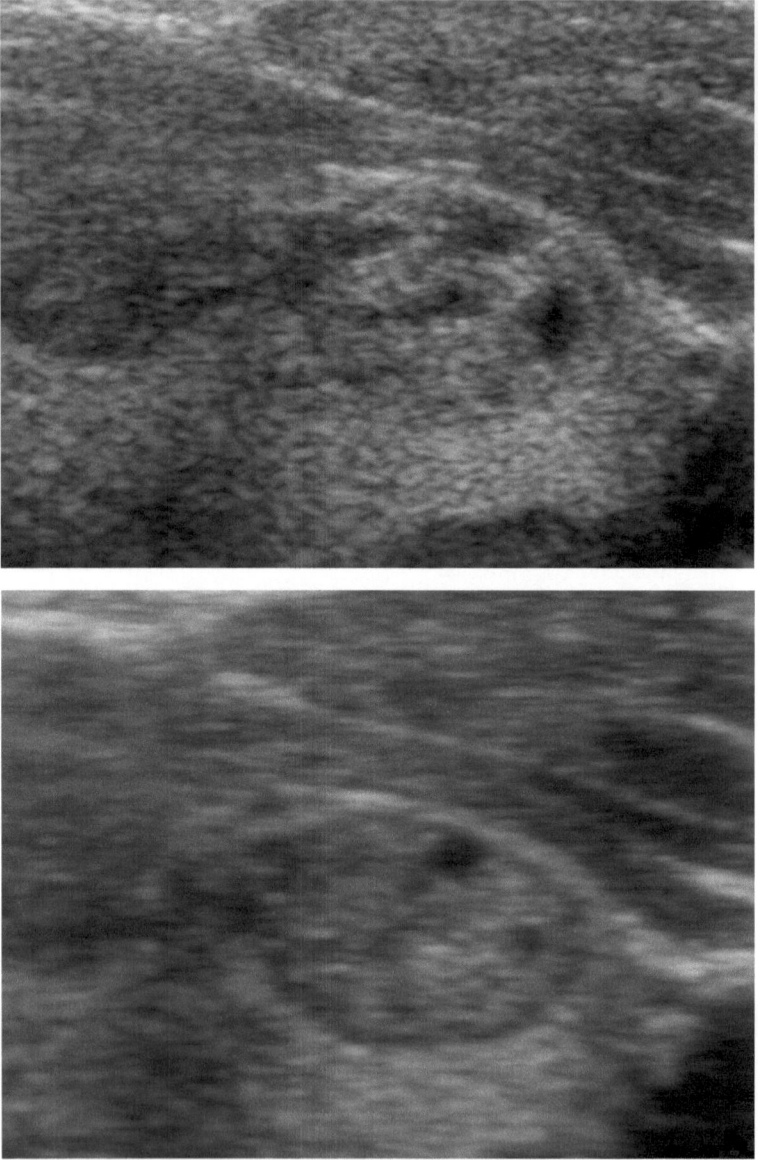

Figure 2.2: A benign thyroid nodule in conventional imaging mode (top) demonstrates acoustic speckle. Spatial compounding mode (bottom) dramatically reduces speckle, improves border definition and contrast resolution and generally enhances overall lesion conspicuity. An occasional unwelcome consequence of spatial image compounding is a degree of blurring as well as appreciable reduction in temporal resolution.

Chapter 3

Attenuation Artifacts

> Attenuation artifacts occur where attenuation is either greater or lesser than expected in some parts of the image. These artifacts are very common and occur in a range of imaging situations.

As ultrasound propagates through the human body, its intensity progressively reduces. This reduction in intensity is known as attenuation. The underlying processes that are responsible for attenuation include reflection, absorption, scattering and refraction. The rate of attenuation affecting ultrasound beams in clinical imaging is truly catastrophic. Consider the following example:

> On average, ultrasound attenuates at approximately 0.5 dB for every MHz of transducer frequency for every 1cm of travel. Let's suppose the sonographer is scanning the liver using a 6MHz transducer set at 10cm depth (20cm total travel path). The total attenuation would be $(0.5 \times 6 \times 20)dB = 60dB$. This represents a ratio of initial to received intensity of 1,000,000:1. In other words, the received echo is only one millionth of the intensity it would have been in the absence of attenuation!

Ultrasound machines compensate for the reduced intensity of echoes arriving from deeper regions of the body by automatic amplification algorithms (automatic gain compensation). These techniques work well when the insonated region contains tissues of uniform attenuation rate. However, the attenuation rates vary enormously between tissues of different types. Such variations of attenuation lead to a range of artifacts. Less than expected attenuation leads to **enhancement** artifacts whereas greater than expected attenuation leads to varying degrees of **acoustic shadowing**.

Types of attenuation artifact

1   Enhancement

- Distal acoustic enhancement

- Focal zone banding

2   Shadowing

- Total acoustic shadowing

- Dirty shadowing

- Dropout

- Venetian blind (stripy) shadowing

- Partial shadowing

- Edge shadowing

- Anisotropic dropout

3.1 Distal acoustic enhancement

Also known as

Posterior acoustic enhancement. The term "distal" is preferable to "posterior" because the direction of the enhancement artifact is not necessarily in the posterior direction.

Causative mechanisms

A structure of low attenuation is present within the field of view adjacent to a structure of normal or high attenuation.

Which system assumptions have been breached?

The assumption that attenuation rate is constant.

Typical appearance

A band of increased echogenicity beyond a region of low attenuation. Always along the lines of sight.

Common misconceptions

A common misconception is that an enhancing structure always represents fluid. While it is true that fluid-filled structures found in the human body (blood, bile, urine, serous fluid, amniotic fluid, pus) are generally low attenuating, solid masses can also demonstrate distal acoustic enhancement. For example a solid tumor in a fatty liver may also produce enhancement.

Can this artifact be reduced, eliminated or circumvented?

The effect of this artifact on the image can be somewhat reduced by use of gain and TGC settings, but at the expense of surrounding tissue echogenicity. Spatial compounding tends to reduce the effect of enhancement although the artifact will still be present. Changing the angle of approach will change the direction of enhancement, allowing assessment of the soft tissue regions previously affected by enhancement.

Is this artifact diagnostically useful?

Yes. Enhancement is a one of the diagnostic criteria for cystic lesions. For example, the definition of a simple cyst is: an anechoic, round or oval, smooth walled, avascular structure with distal acoustic enhancement. Enhancement can assist in identification of small cysts because the artifact is larger than the causative structure and is therefore easy to appreciate in the image. Enhancement can also be helpful in determining the probability of a mass being fluid-filled or solid.

It is important to keep in mind that many normal anatomical structures will cause enhancement, including blood vessels, gallbladder, urinary bladder and ovarian follicles.

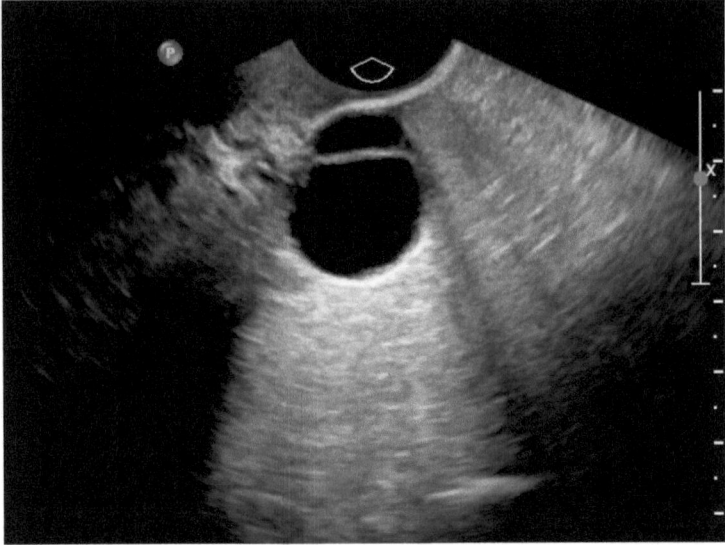

Figure 3.1: The most common examples of distal acoustic enhancement are found in association with simple cysts such as liver cysts, renal cysts or in this case ovarian cysts.

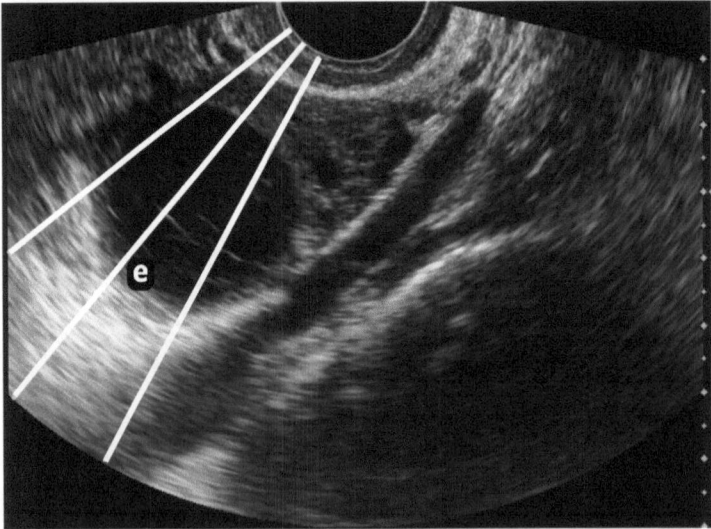

Figure 3.2: Acoustic enhancement (e) beyond a hemorrhagic ovarian cyst on transvaginal scan performed with a tightly curved array. Note that the direction of the enhancement is along the lines of sight, not necessarily vertical in the image.

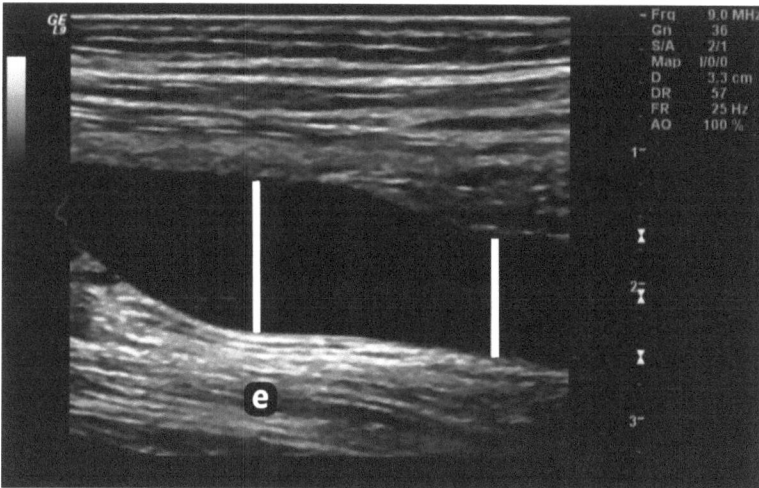

Figure 3.3: Superficial vein in longitudinal section demonstrates distal acoustic enhancement. The enhancement (e) is more pronounced where the vessel diameter is greater (left line) because the region of low attenuation is greater along the lines of sight at that location.

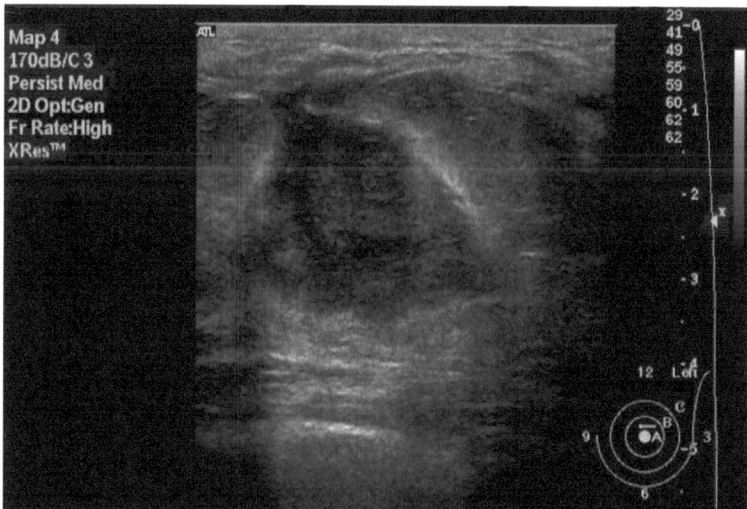

Figure 3.4: This hypoechoic heterogeneous breast mass with distal acoustic enhancement represents a breast abscess. The abscess cavity contains pus with thick particulate debris which can appear on ultrasound as hypoechoic or echogenic internal material. The abscess contents are of lower attenuation than surrounding soft tissue, leading to enhancement.

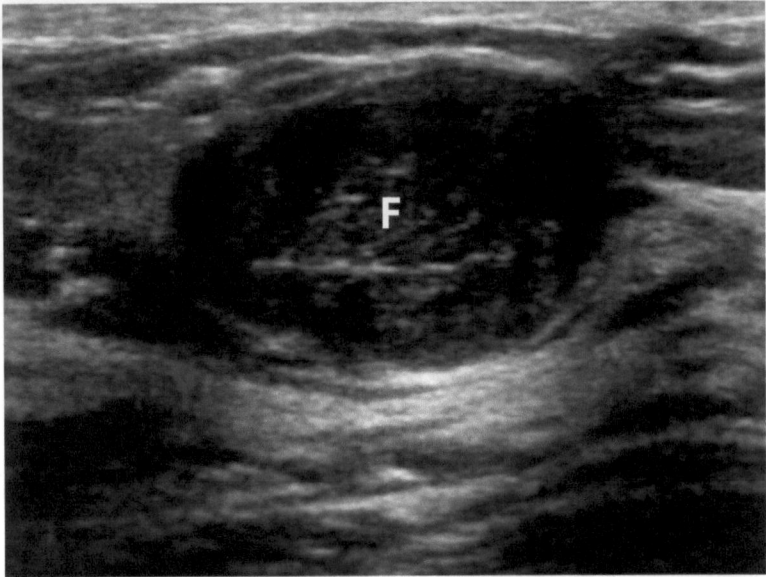

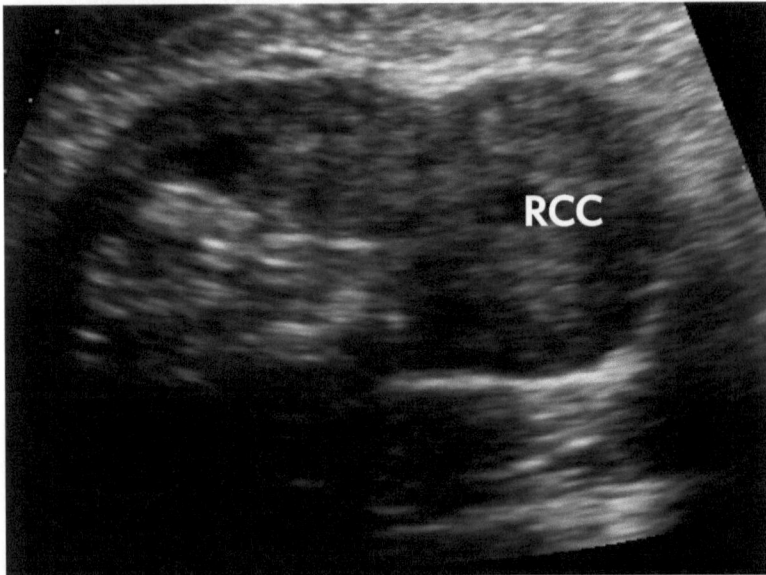

Figure 3.5: A wide range of solid masses can demonstrate enhancement when surrounded by higher attenuation tissue. The examples above include fibroadenoma of the breast (F) and renal cell carcinoma (RCC).

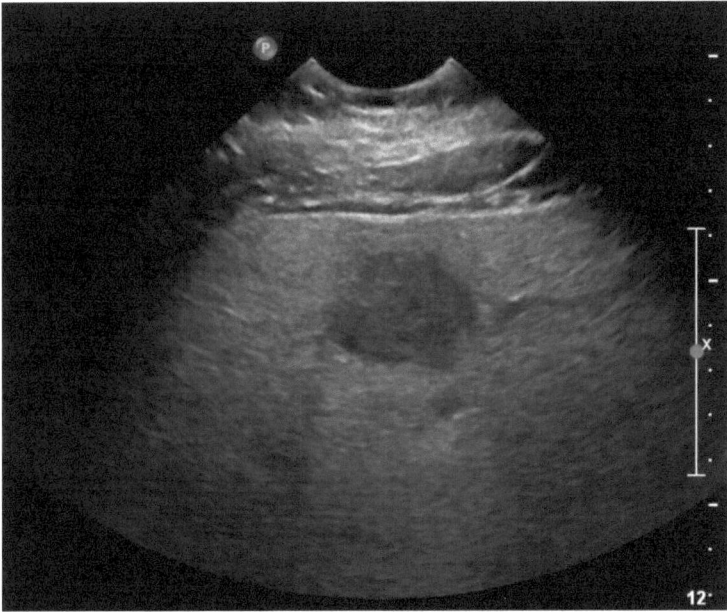

Figure 3.6: Liver hemangioma with distal acoustic enhancement on the background of an attenuating fatty liver.

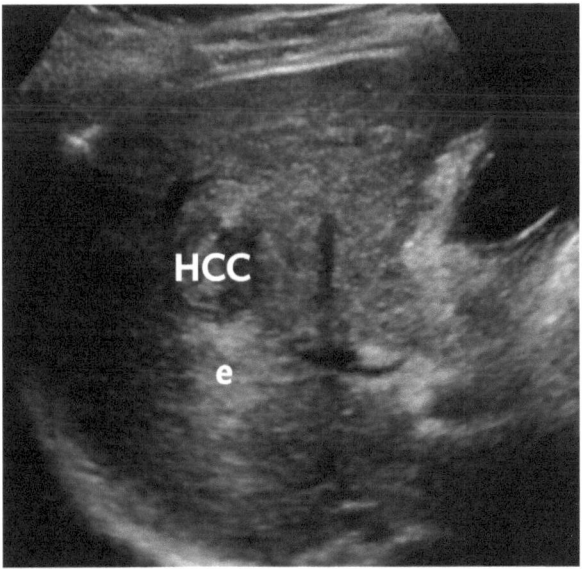

Figure 3.7: Enhancing hepatocellular carcinoma (HCC) in a dense, attenuating cirrhotic liver.

3.2 Focal zone banding

Also known as

Banding

Causative mechanisms

The intensity of ultrasound and the resultant amplitude of returning echoes are greatest at the focal point. Sometimes this leads to a band of increased brightness in the focal region.

Typical appearance

A horizontal band of increased echogenicity at the level of the focal zone.

Can this artifact be reduced, eliminated or circumvented?

The artifact can usually be completely eliminated with the adjustment of time gain compensation (TGC).

Is this artifact diagnostically useful?

No.

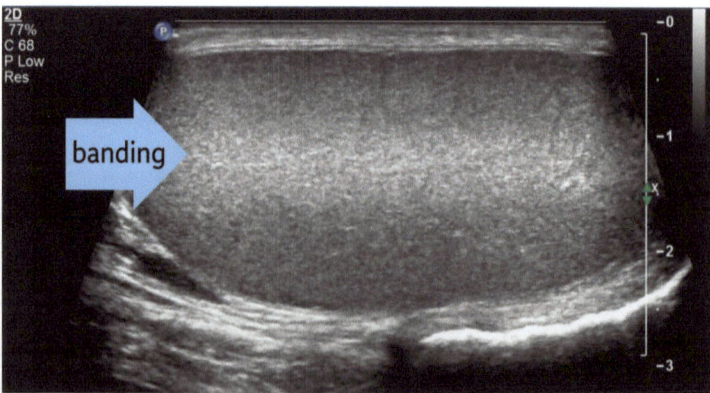

Figure 3.8: Normal testis demonstrating a horizontal band of increased echogenicity at the level of the focal zone.

3.3 Total distal acoustic shadowing

Also known as

Complete shadowing or clean shadowing.

Causative mechanisms

A structure of high attenuation is present within the field of view adjacent to a structure of normal or low attenuation. Attenuation can be due to reflection, scattering, absorption, refraction or any combination of these factors. Ultrasound either does not penetrate into the causative structure at all or it penetrates but gets rapidly absorbed. This leads to a complete absence of echo information from regions beyond the causative structure.

Which system assumptions have been breached?

The assumption that the attenuation rate is constant.

Typical appearance

Anechoic shadow beyond the causative structure. Always along the lines of sight. Total shadowing requires the causative structure to be larger than the beam dimensions (beamwidth and slice thickness), otherwise parts of the beam bypass the attenuating structure and echoes are produced beyond it.

Common misconceptions

It is a common misconception that the causative structure is always hard and solid, such as bone, gallstone, calcification, etc. Gas can also produce total shadowing. Soft tissues of high attenuation (fibrous tissues), anisotropic and refracting tissues (such as vessel walls and ligaments) investigated at acute angles also cast acoustic shadows.

Can this artifact be reduced, eliminated or circumvented?

This artifact cannot be completely eliminated. If the causative structure is relatively small, spatial compounding can confine the shadowing effect to a smaller region just beyond the causative structure. Beam steering can sometimes allow investigation of tissues beyond the shadowing structure.

To fully interrogate the region within the shadow usually requires a new acoustic window. This may not always be technically possible.

Is this artifact diagnostically useful?

The presence of shadowing is a useful diagnostic criterion for biliary or renal calculi and calcifications. For example, the definition of a gallstone within the gallbladder is that of an echogenic, mobile, shadowing mass. In some circumstances, shadowing may be more apparent than the causative structure itself. This improves the operator's ability to find a subtle mass, for example a small breast malignancy or a foreign body.

It is important to keep in mind that small structures such as small gallstones or kidney stones may not demonstrate shadowing if the size of the object is smaller than the beamwidth. To demonstrate or accentuate shadows from small structures, sonographers should use the highest frequency transducer possible and turn off spatial compounding.

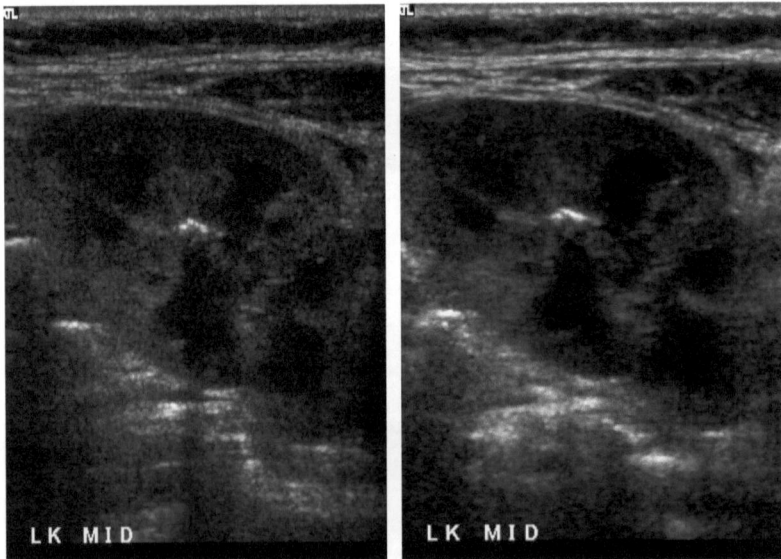

Figure 3.9: In this example, a small renal calculus casts an acoustic shadow when interrogated in conventional imaging mode without spatial compounding (left image). With spatial compounding turned on (right image), the shadow is much less apparent.

Unfortunately acoustic shadowing may sometimes mask regions of pathology.

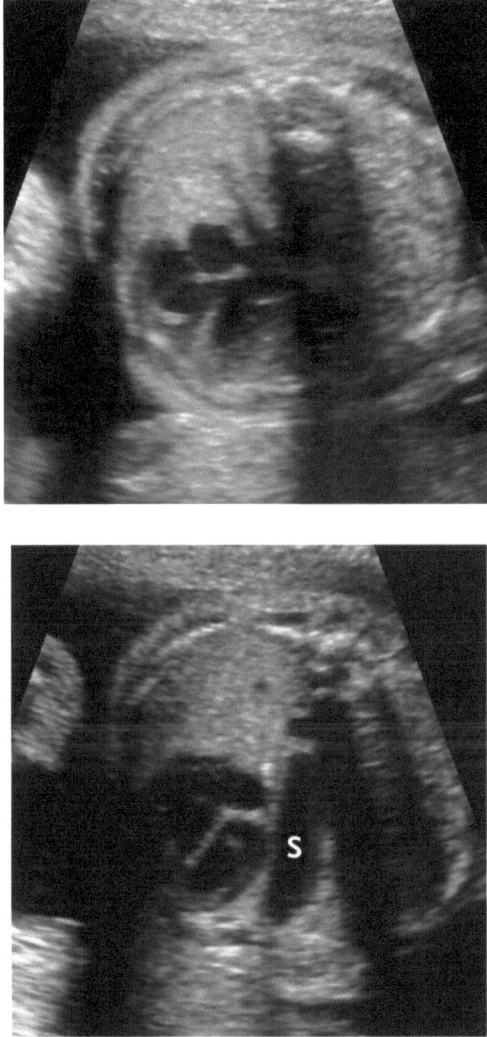

Figure 3.10: (Top) A transverse view of the fetal chest is shown. The sonographer noted an abnormal cardiac axis. The cause is not evident in this image because an important diagnostic clue is hidden in the shadow from the fetal spine. (Bottom) A different angle of approach revealed the fetal stomach (s) adjacent to the heart in this fetus with a congenital diaphragmatic hernia.

Total acoustic shadowing: examples

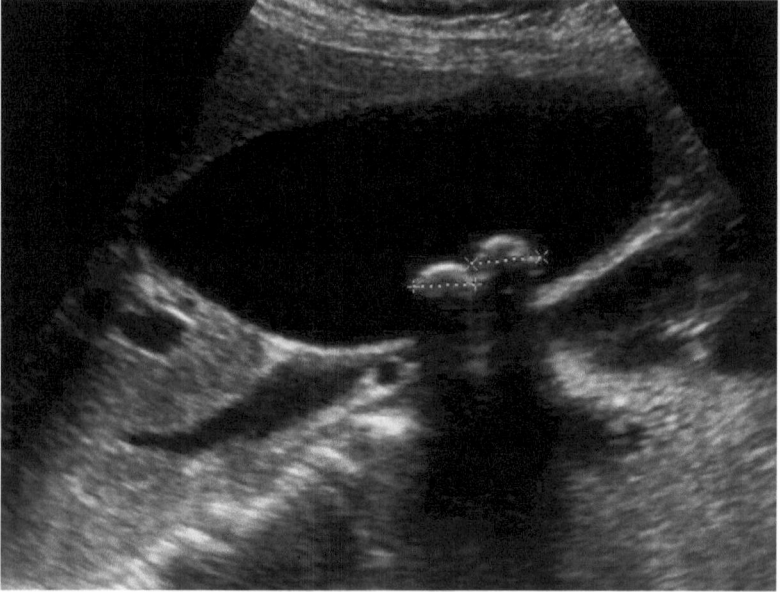

Figure 3.11: Classic appearance of acoustic shadowing associated with gallstones.

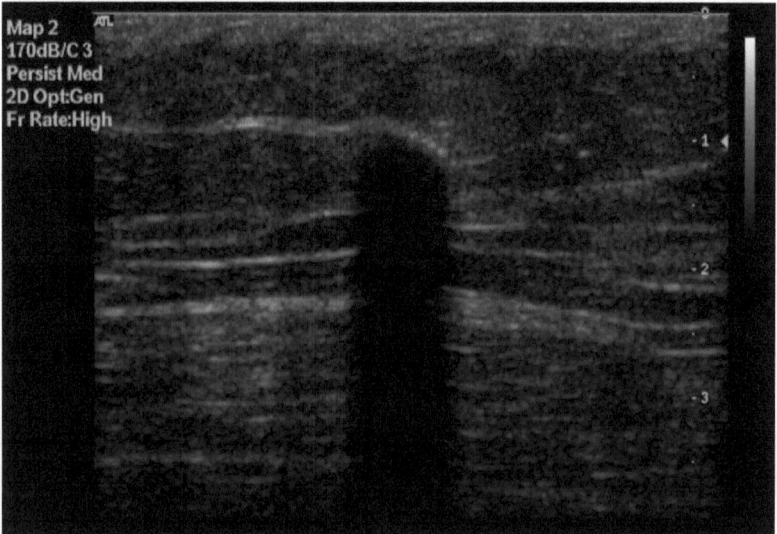

Figure 3.12: A skin calcification scanned in conventional mode demonstrates total acoustic shadowing.

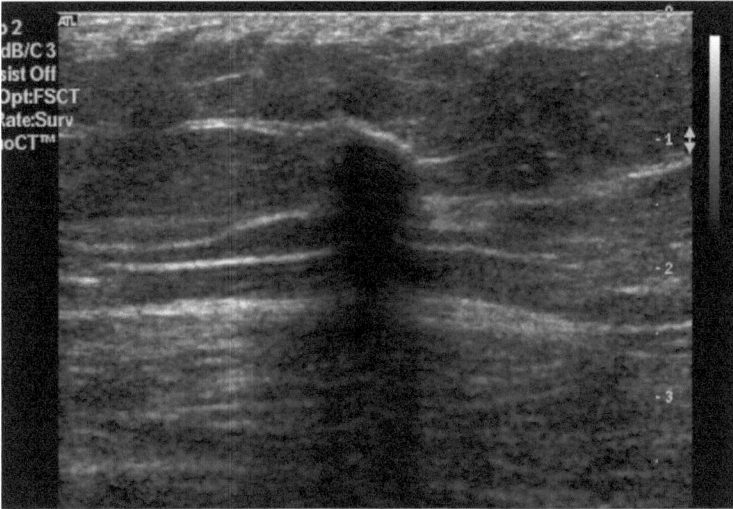

Figure 3.13: The mass in Figure 3.12 has been scanned in spatial compounding mode. Now it casts a clean central shadow surrounded by a dirty shadow.

In spatial compounding a smaller mass may produce multiple shadows.

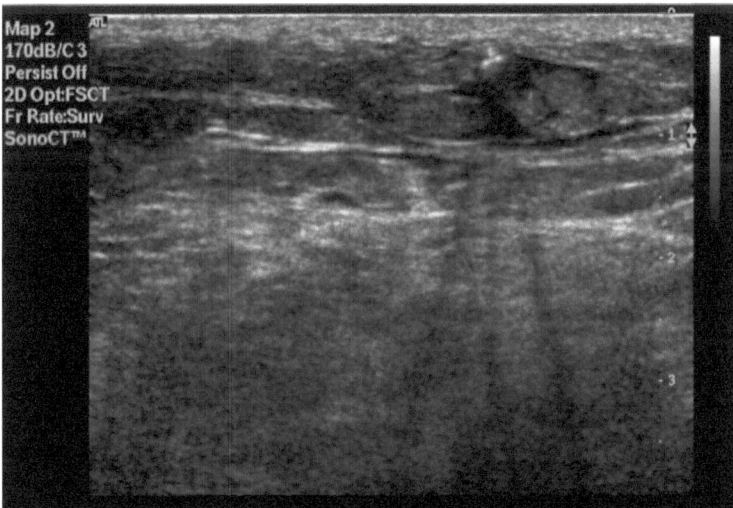

Figure 3.14: A hypodermic needle is imaged in transverse view using spatial compounding. The needle casts acoustic shadows along multiple lines of sight. If spatial compounding was turned off, only the middle vertical shadow would remain. This artifact has previously been described as the "Sputnik" artifact in recognition of the artifact's similarity to the first artificial satellite.

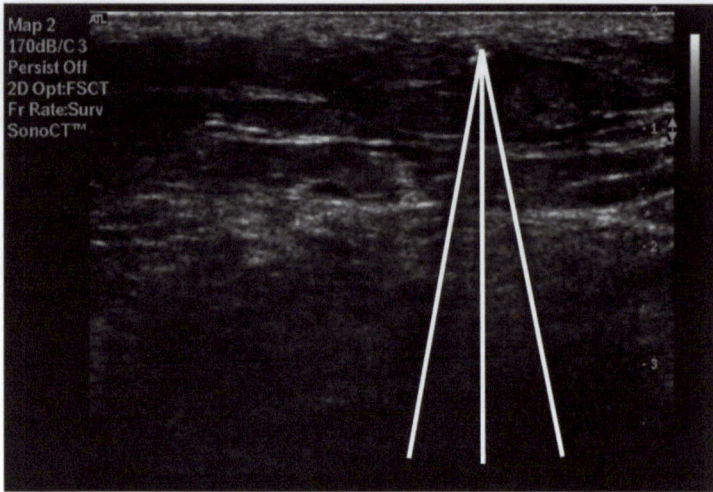

Figure 3.15: The same image as Figure 3.14 with the multiple shadows highlighted.

Shadowing can also be important in 3D imaging.

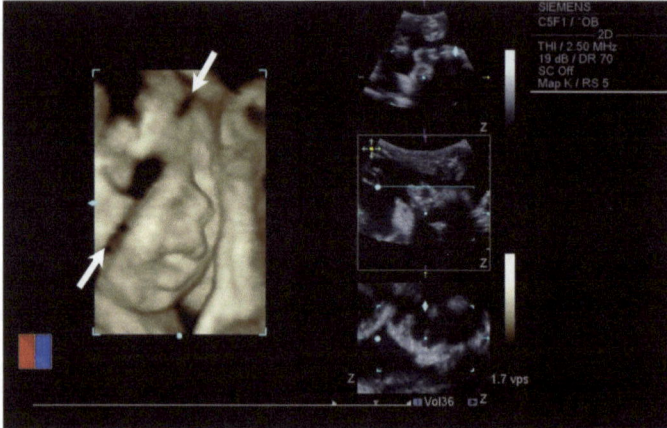

Figure 3.16: All artifacts that affect ultrasound imaging in 2D (sectional) imaging also affect 3D imaging. Some artifacts can be accentuated in 3D. It is also possible that the artifact may be innocuous on multiplanar reformats (MPR), but be very pronounced in volume renderings. This image demonstrates a surface volume rendering of the fetal face. A large shadow is seen diagonally crossing the face (highlighted by the arrows). The causative structure is the fetal arm which is not seen in this projection of the volume rendering.

3.4 Dirty shadowing

Also known as

Incomplete shadowing

Causative mechanisms

As with total acoustic shadowing, a structure of high attenuation is present within the field of view adjacent to a structure of normal or low attenuation. Ultrasound penetrates into the causative structure and produces some echoes but is highly attenuated in the process.

Which system assumptions have been breached?

The assumption that the attenuation rate is constant.

Typical appearance

Hypoechoic shadow beyond the causative structure. Always along the lines of sight.

Can this artifact be reduced, eliminated or circumvented?

If the dirty shadowing is minor, adjustments in TGC and gain may allow the operator to investigate the tissues beyond the causative structure. Some machines also allow the operator to change lateral gain compensation or the system may have a built-in automated gain compensation algorithm. If the dirty shadowing is severe, a new acoustic window must be used to interrogate the distal tissues. This may not always be technically possible.

Is this artifact diagnostically useful?

Most of the time, this artifact is a nuisance and is not diagnostically helpful.

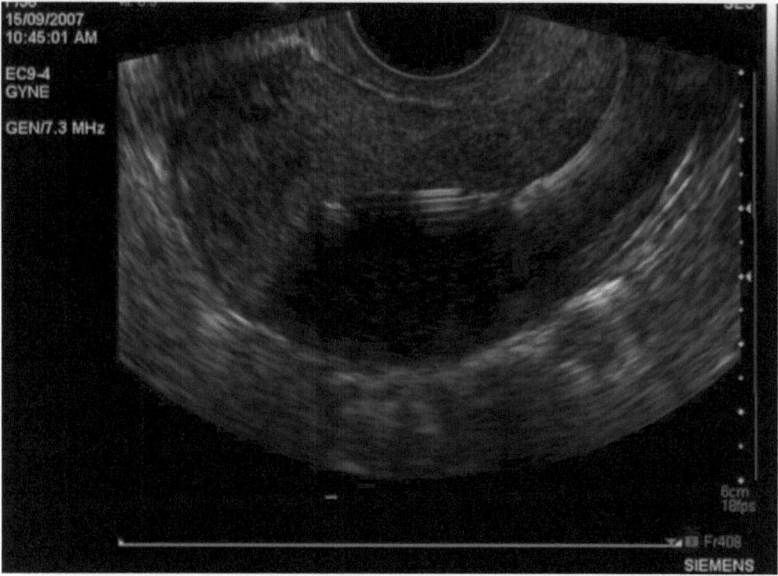

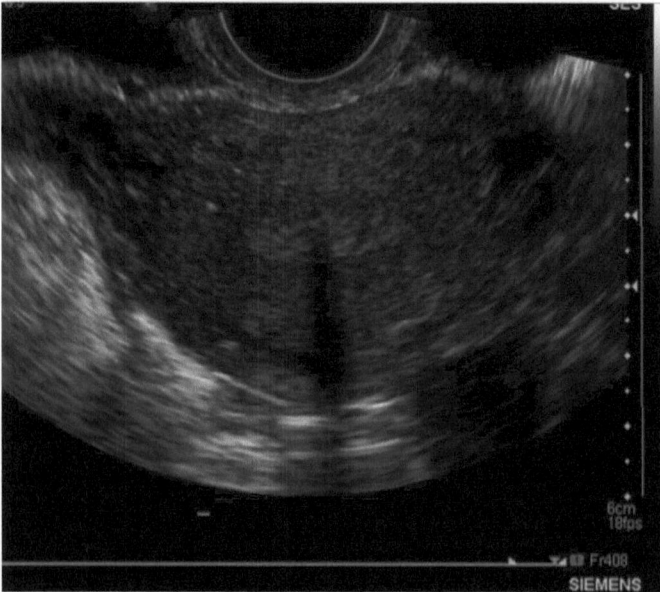

Figure 3.17: Mirena intrauterine contraceptive device (IUCD) in longitudinal (top) and transverse (bottom) section may cast complete or dirty shadow depending on the beam dimensions at the location of the device.

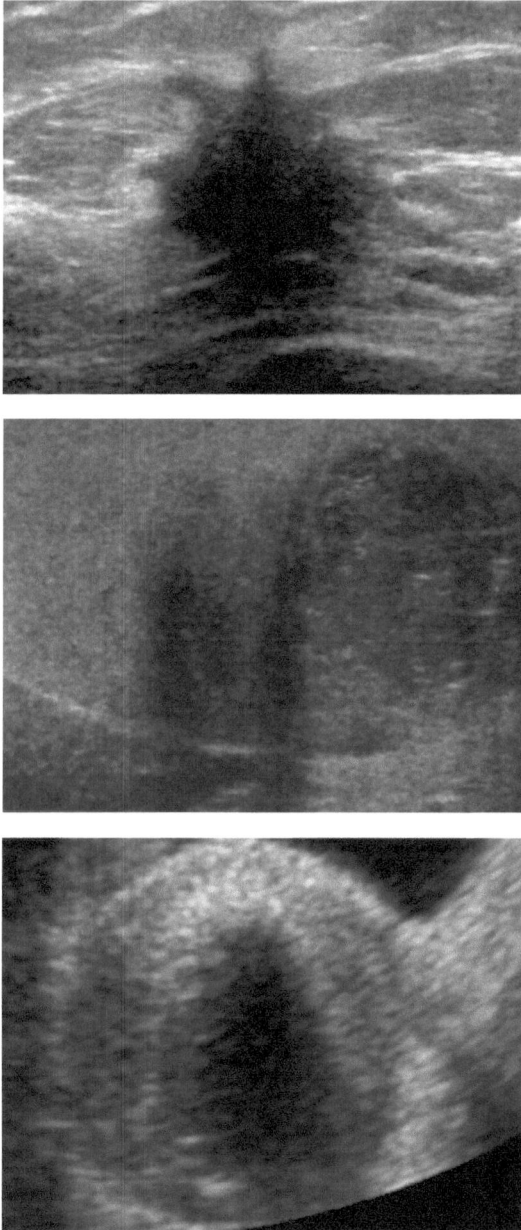

Figure 3.18: A wide range of benign or malignant masses can produce dirty shadowing. The examples here include: spiculated malignant breast tumor (top), infiltrative testicular seminoma (center) and ovarian dermoid containing hair (bottom).

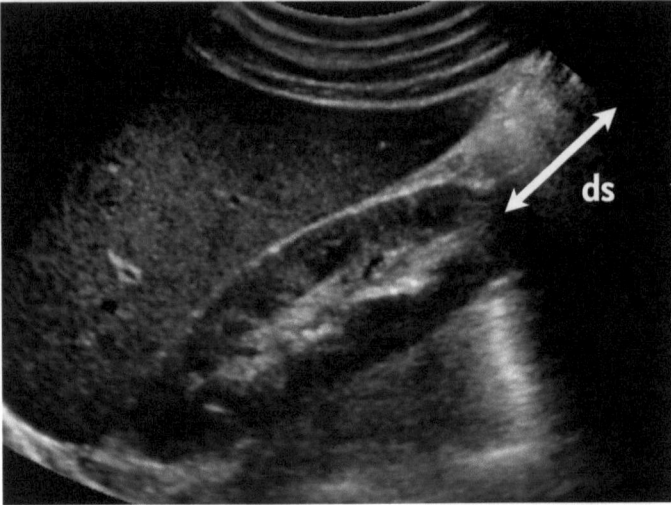

Figure 3.19: Gas is a common cause of dirty shadowing. In this image, bowel gas casts a dirty shadow (ds) over the lower pole of the right kidney. In order to evaluate this area and exclude an exophytic renal mass, the operator must use a different approach.

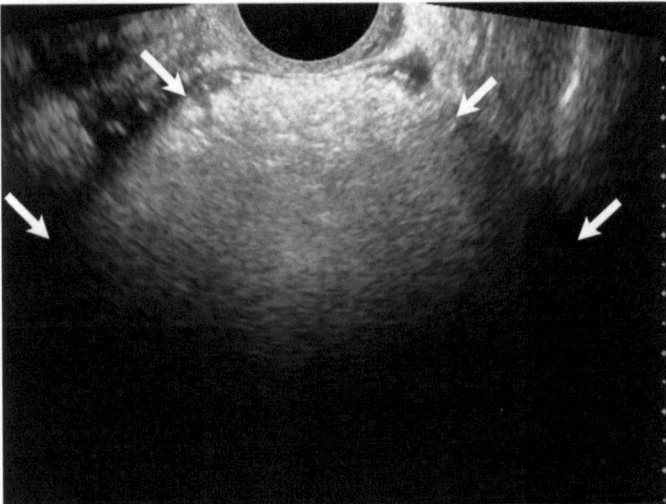

Figure 3.20: This large attenuating ovarian dermoid could easily be mistaken for a loop of bowel. The diagnostic clues which allowed differentiation of this ovarian neoplasm from bowel included: 1) the large diameter of the mass and 2) the lack of peristalsis.

3.5 Dropout

Causative mechanisms

Dropout, like all forms of acoustic shadowing, is caused by an attenuating structure in the field of view. Ultrasound penetrates the causative structure and produces some echoes but is attenuated in the process. Dropout may also occur with the use of small apertures (focus close to the transducer) because the ultrasound beam will have wide divergence in the far field resulting in rapid loss of intensity.

Which system assumptions have been breached?

Assumption that attenuation rate is constant.

Typical appearance

Hypoechoic or anechoic region beyond the causative structure. Always along the lines of sight.

Can this artifact be reduced, eliminated or circumvented?

Some forms of drop-out can be eliminated with the use of a more favorable acoustic window. Other strategies for reducing dropout include: 1) increasing gain or TGC settings, 2) reducing the operating frequency of the transducer or switching to a lower frequency transducer to improve penetration and 3) switching from harmonic to fundamental frequency imaging.

Is this artifact diagnostically useful?

Most of the time, this artifact is a nuisance and is not diagnostically helpful.

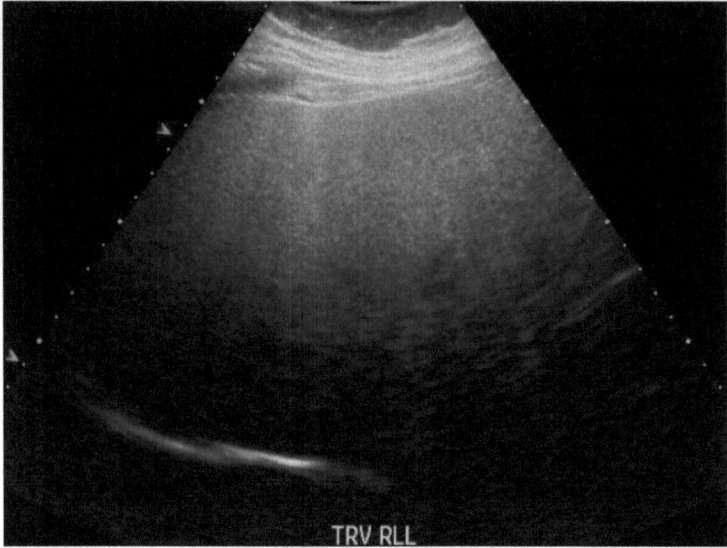

Figure 3.21: Diminished penetration is seen in this patient with advanced steatosis.

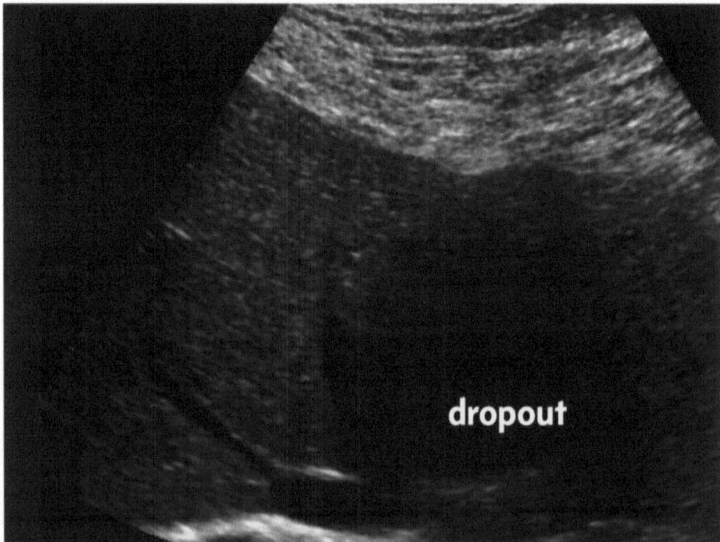

Figure 3.22: Figures 3.22 and 3.23 demonstrate the same normal liver scanned through the subxiphoid epigastric window. In this image, penetration is compromised due to a poor acoustic window (the xiphoid is partially obstructing the acoustic window).

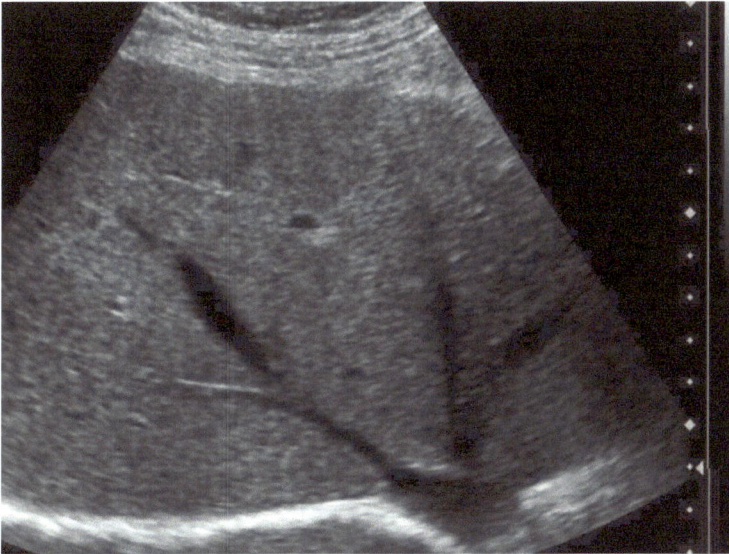

Figure 3.23: Adjustment of the acoustic window has yielded an improved diagnostic image.

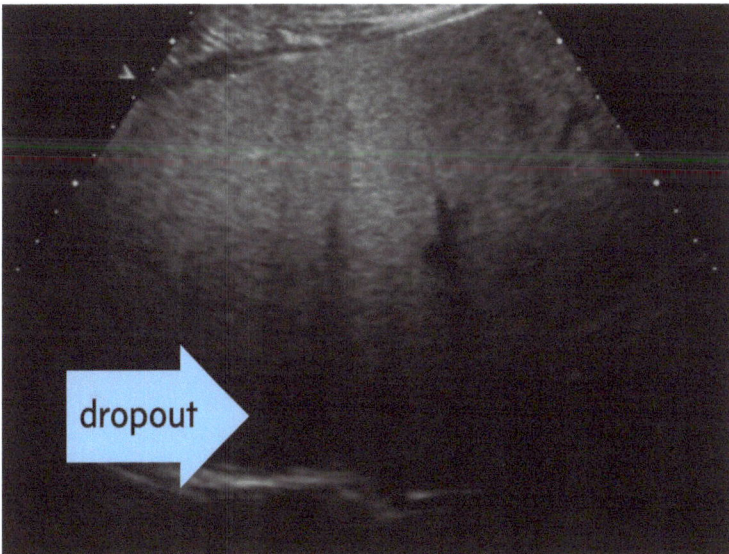

Figure 3.24: Dropout artifact is seen in the liver of a patient with chronic liver disease when the examination is performed with a 6C2 transducer at 4MHz. As shown in Figure 3.25, switching to 2.5MHz eliminates dropout but the trade-off is reduction in spatial resolution.

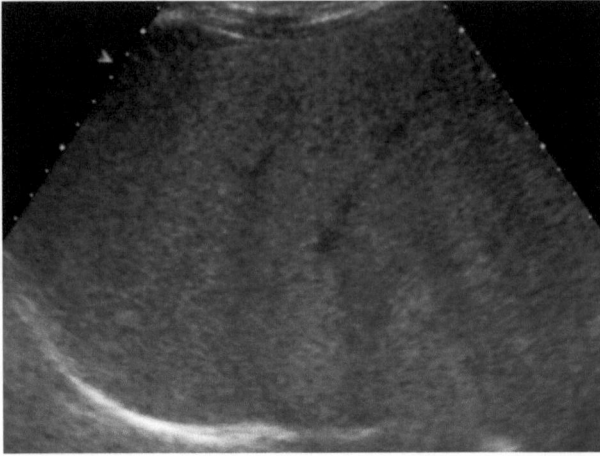

Figure 3.25: Using a lower frequency has eliminated the dropout but the spatial resolution is reduced.

Dropout can also be due to a loss of transducer contact with the patient or absence of acoustic couplant (gel). This cause is usually quite obvious as there is complete lack of any diagnostic information in the image from the transducer surface down.

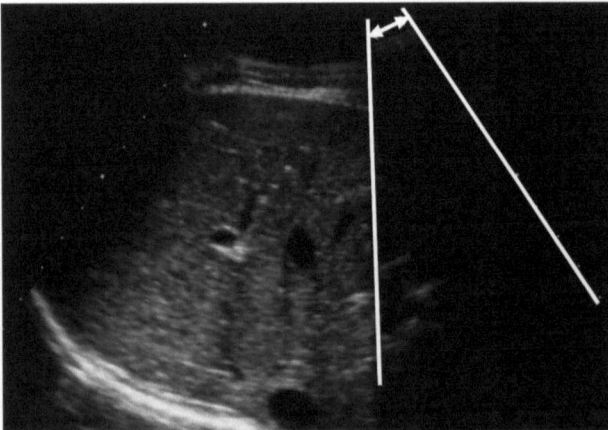

Figure 3.26: When spatial compounding mode is on, some echo information may be gathered in the zone of drop-out from adjacent apertures which are in good contact with the patient. The double arrow in this image highlights the zone of no transducer contact.

In the images below the dropout artifact is seen below the level of the portal vein in a normal patient. The region of the portal vein is attenuating due to the presence of fibrous tissue which binds together the portal triad.

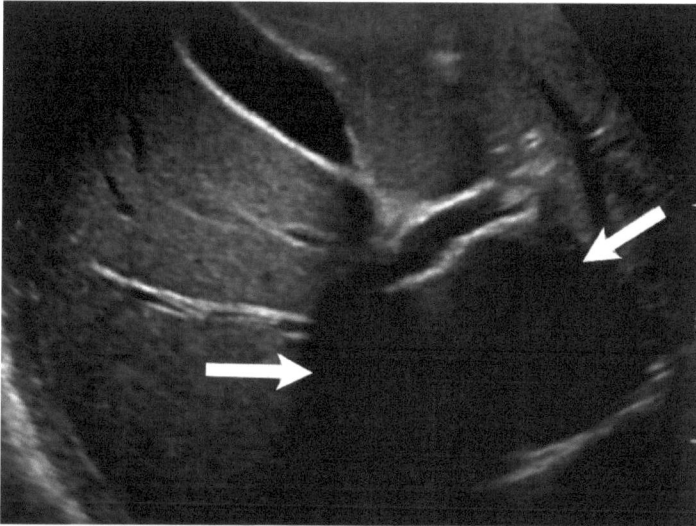

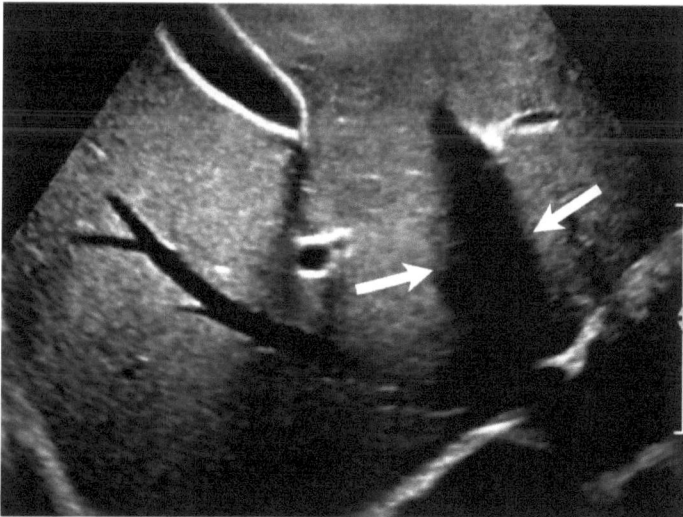

Figure 3.27: Dropout artifact is seen below the level of the portal vein in a normal patient.

Inflammatory reactions or edema in subcutaneous fat often result in increased tissue echogenicity and increased attenuation (see example in Figures 3.28 and 3.29).

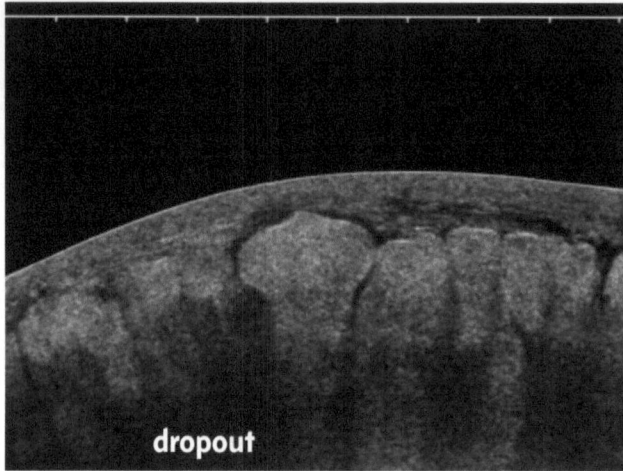

Figure 3.28: A region of acute cellulitis was scanned using a high frequency linear array transducer. The dropout artifact was visualized beyond a depth of 2-3cm.

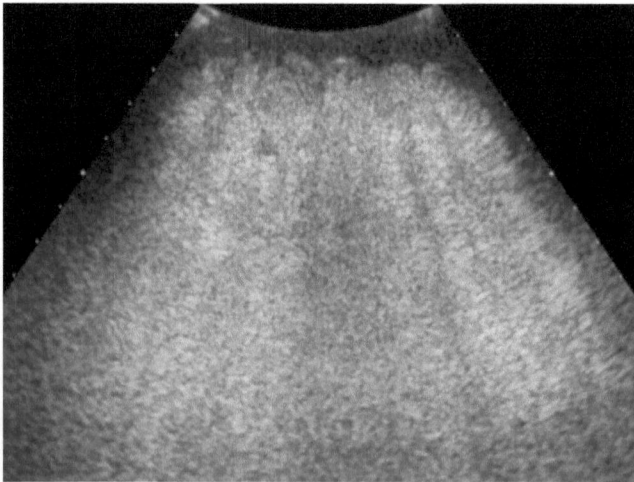

Figure 3.29: To exclude a deeper collection, the sonographer switched to a low frequency curvilinear transducer which allowed penetration to a depth exceeding 10cm.

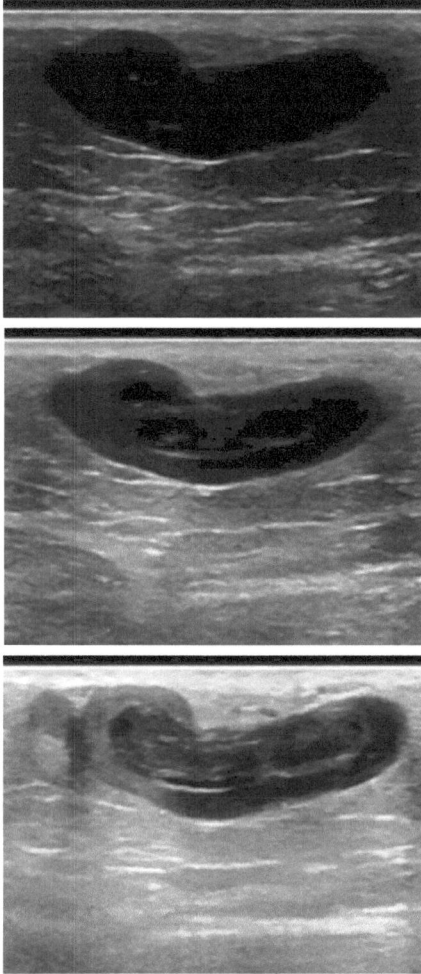

Figure 3.30: Dropout can also occur due to an inappropriate level of gain or TGC set by the operator. The top image shows an apparently anechoic superficial vein. Progressive increase in gain reveals some low-level echoes in the middle image and eventually a large non-occlusive heterogeneous thrombus is seen in the bottom image. Under most imaging circumstances, using slightly conservative gain results in improvement of contrast resolution. In some ultrasound applications, such as vascular ultrasound, sonographers may be compelled to reduce gain and dynamic range more aggressively in order to achieve a high level of contrast and eliminate artifacts that contaminate the vessel lumen. Unfortunately, reduction of gain and dynamic range is also associated with loss of sensitivity and may lead to dropout of real echoes as demonstrated in these images.

Focusing has a major impact on the beam intensity in various parts of the field of view. When the operator positions the transmit focus close to the transducer, the system is forced to use small apertures that produce beams with a high degree of far-field divergence. This results in a dramatic loss of beam and echo intensity.

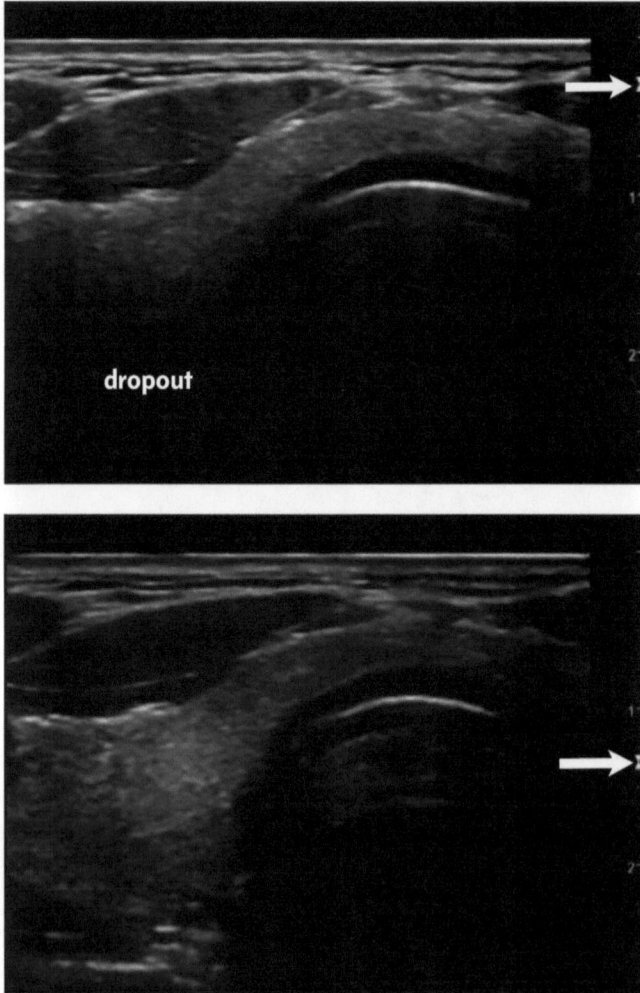

Figure 3.31: These images show a normal thyroid gland. The upper image was obtained with a focal zone inappropriately positioned close to the transducer (arrow). Dropout is seen beyond a 15mm depth. Simple re-positioning of the focal zone to a deeper location eliminates dropout in this case (lower image).

3.6 Venetian-blind shadowing

Also known as

Stripy shadowing.

Causative mechanisms

The insonated tissue contains multiple adjacent small regions of high and low attenuation.

Which system assumptions have been breached?

The assumption that the attenuation rate is constant.

Typical appearance

Hypoechoic or anechoic stripes along the lines of sight.

Can this artifact be reduced, eliminated or circumvented?

This artifact cannot be eliminated.

Is this artifact diagnostically useful?

Yes. This artifact is typical of some pathologies, for example uterine adenomyosis. The artifact is also commonly seen in association with subcutaneous edema or lymphedema but is not helpful in this instance because the combination of edema and shadowing prevents investigation of deeper structures relevant to the patient's clinical condition such as the deep veins.

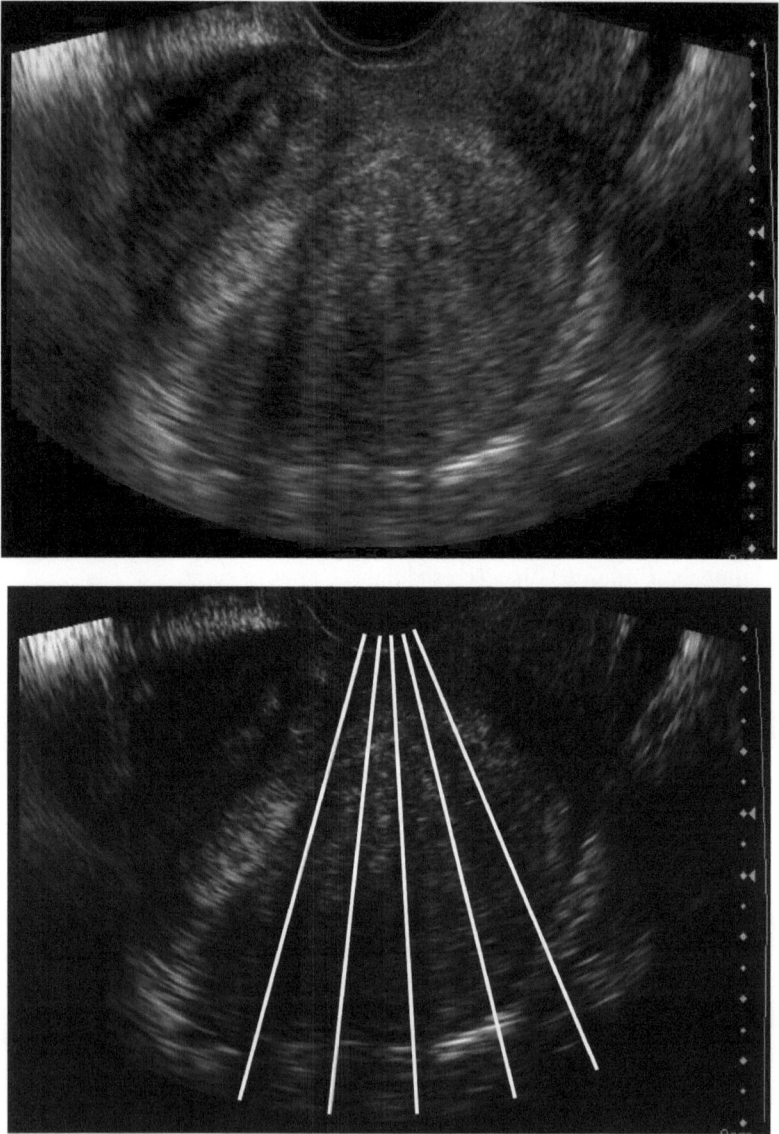

Figure 3.32: Venetian blind shadowing is a classic finding in uterine adeno-myosis.

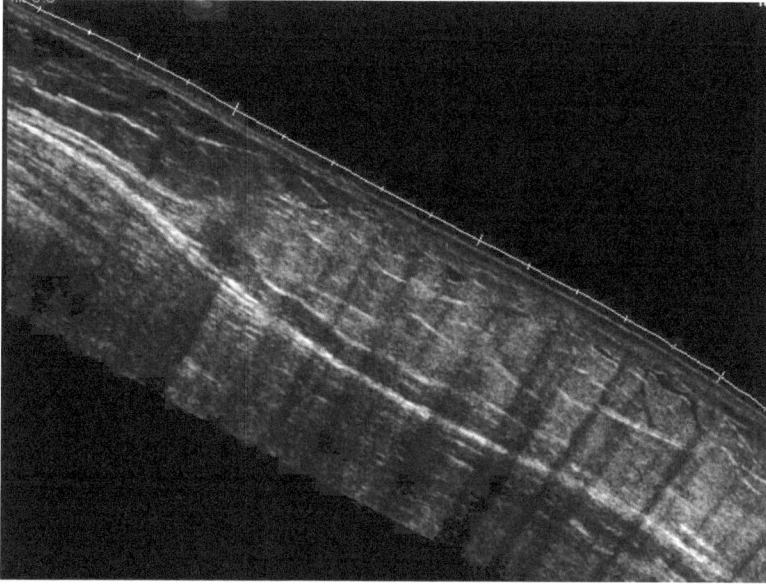

Figure 3.33: Panoramic view of the lower extremity in a patient with cellulitis demonstrates Venetian blind shadowing associated with the region of inflammation and swelling.

3.7 Partial shadowing

Causative mechanisms

Partial shadowing is similar to dropout and represents a range of minor attenuation problems caused by poor acoustic windows, tissue nonuniformity, scarring, attenuating structures projecting into the slice-thickness plane of the transducer and others.

Which system assumptions have been breached?

The assumption that the attenuation rate is constant.

Typical appearance

Variable loss of intensity manifesting as reduced tissue echogenicity.

Can this artifact be reduced, eliminated or circumvented?

The operator may be able to find a more favorable acoustic window.

Is this artifact diagnostically useful?

No. Partial shadowing is not useful.

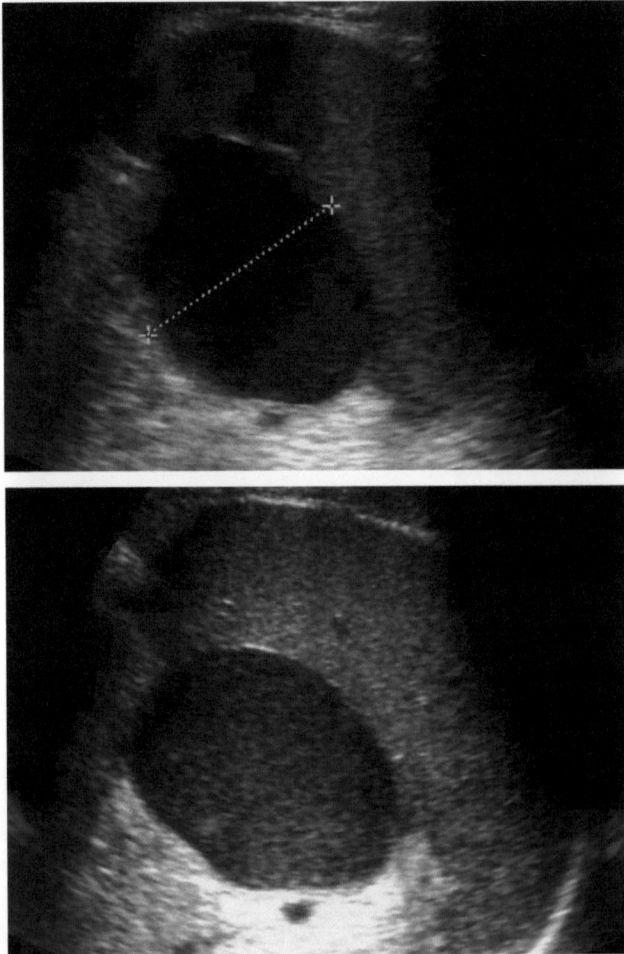

Figure 3.34: This pancreatic pseudocyst appears artifactually anechoic in the top image because the transducer is partially resting on the rib. A small movement of the transducer into the intercostal window reveals the echogenic particulate nature of the fluid collection.

3.8 Edge shadowing

Also known as

Edge effect, refraction shadowing, refraction edge shadowing or edge defocusing.

Causative mechanisms

The cause of edge shadowing is a combination of reflection and refraction at the margin of a well defined mass. These factors lead to defocusing of the beam, loss of beam intensity and corresponding appearance of shadowing beyond the causative margin.

Which system assumptions have been breached?

All of the following assumptions are breached: 1) speed of sound is constant, 2) sound travels in a straight line and 3) attenuation rate is constant.

Typical appearance

Shadow originating from the margin of a well defined cystic or solid structure.

Common misconceptions

Edge shadowing is not only associated with cystic masses but can also be associated with solid masses or normal organ margins (such as the margin of the kidney).

Can this artifact be reduced, eliminated or circumvented?

Edge shadowing can be significantly reduced with the use of spatial compounding. A change in the angle of approach alters the direction of the shadow which allows investigation of regions previously affected by shadowing.

Is this artifact diagnostically useful?

No. This artifact is not useful.

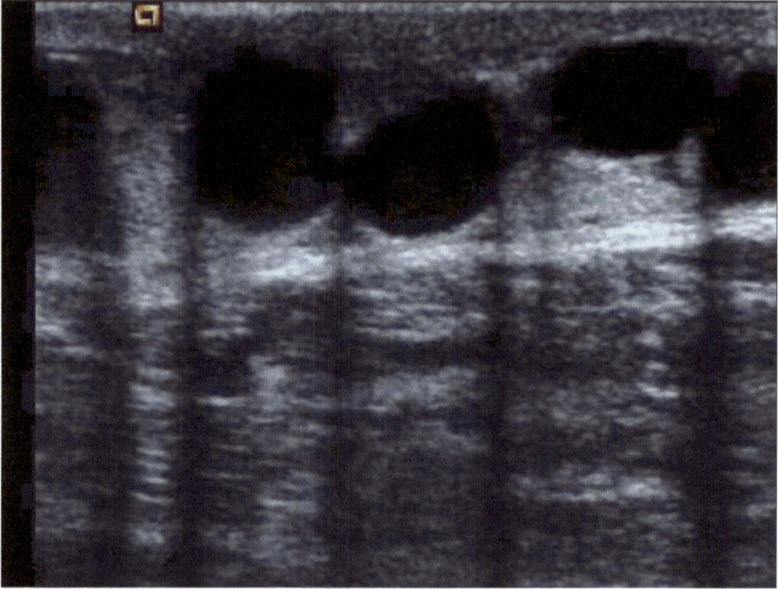

Figure 3.35: A cluster of varicose veins demonstrates multiple edge shadows.

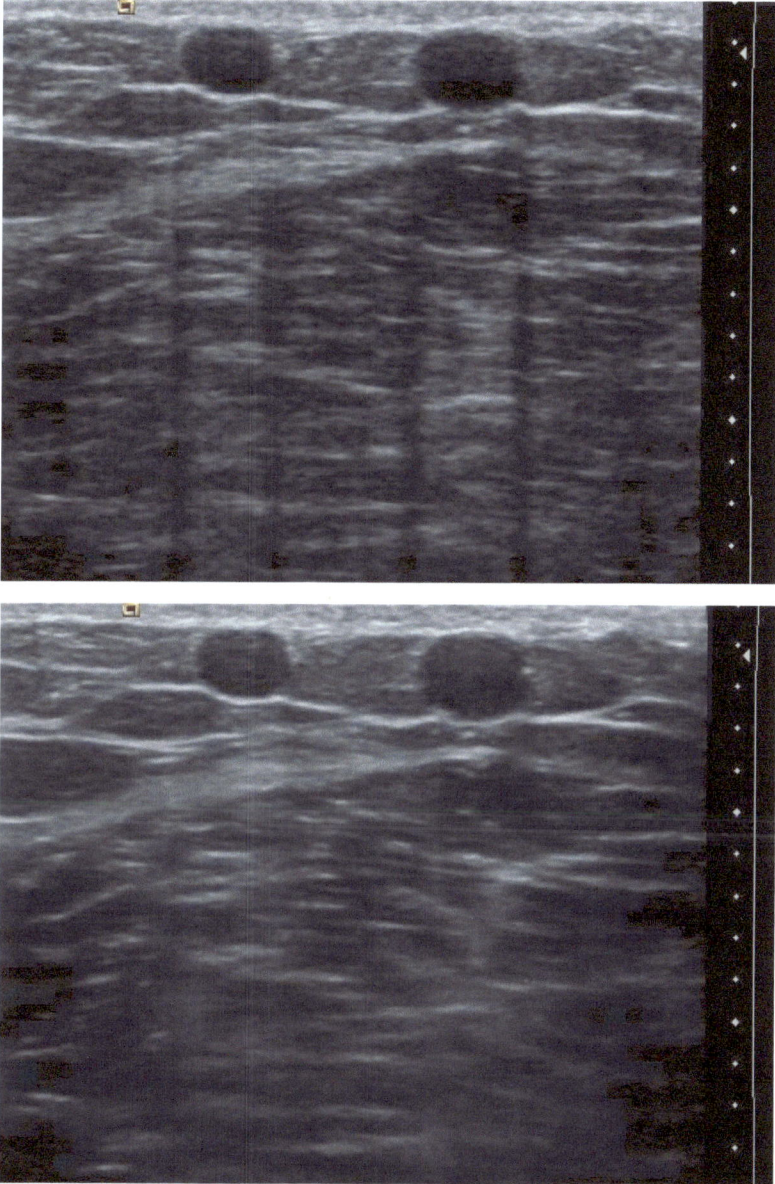

Figure 3.36: The same varicose veins scanned without spatial compounding (top) and with spatial compounding (bottom). Refraction shadowing has been completely eliminated in the compounded image.

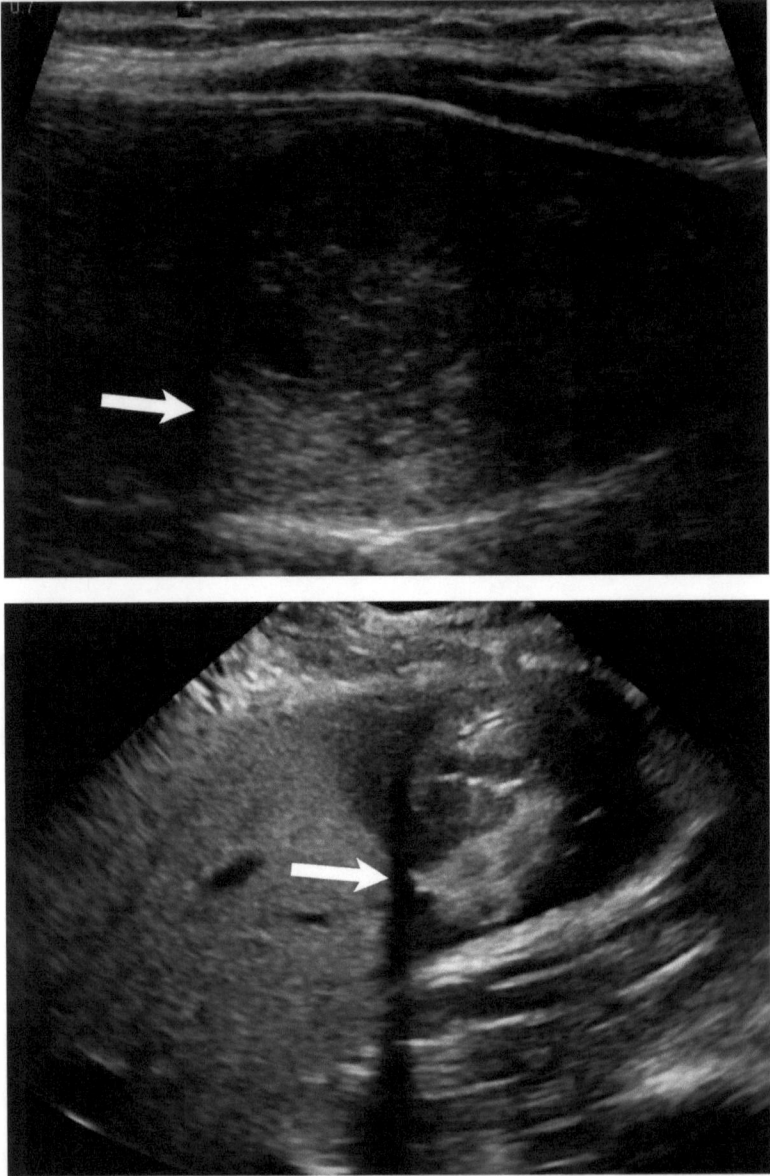

Figure 3.37: Examples of edge shadowing associated with solid masses: thyroid nodule (upper image) and liver metastasis (lower image).

Example showing edge shadowing, dirty shadowing and total shadowing.

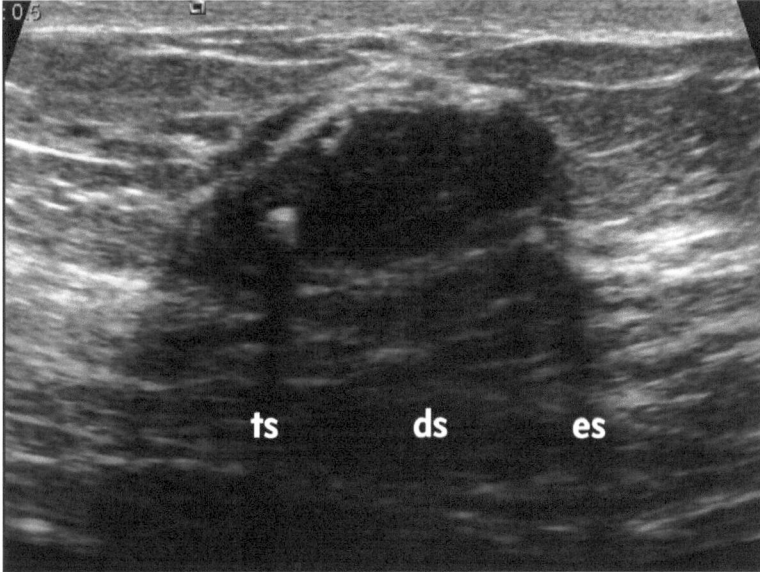

Figure 3.38: In this image of a breast fibroadenoma, nearly all forms of shadowing are present. The internal calcification casts a total shadow (ts), the remainder of the mass causes a dirty shadow (ds) and edge shadowing is also present especially on the right (es).

3.9 Anisotropic dropout

Also known as

Anisotropy.

Causative mechanisms

Anisotropy is due to variable propagation speed across and along striated structures such as muscles, tendons and ligaments.

When an anisotropic structure is interrogated from an angle other than normal (90°) incidence, the incident beam refracts at each interface within the structure which leads to a rapid defocusing effect manifesting as loss of echo amplitude, attenuation and dropout. The problem is well known in musculoskeletal ultrasound.

Which system assumptions have been breached?

All of the following assumptions are breached: 1) speed of sound is constant, 2) sound travels in a straight line and 3) attenuation rate is constant.

Typical appearance

Normal striated appearance of the structure of interest (muscle, tendon, ligament) at normal incidence (90°) but gradual loss of echogenicity at angles less than 90° with complete drop-out at acute angles.

Can this artifact be reduced, eliminated or circumvented?

Yes, this artifact can be eliminated if the region of interest can be scanned at normal incidence by manually angling the transducer, electronic beam-steering or the use of a favorable acoustic window. If a 90° approach is not achievable, anisotropy is difficult to eliminate. Spatial image compounding tends to reduce the effect of anisotropy because some of the beams will interrogate the region of interest at a favorable angle.

Is this artifact diagnostically useful?

No. This artifact is a major problem in musculoskeletal imaging. For example, curved tendons need to be interrogated from a range of angles because some parts of the tendon will always demonstrate dropout. Less experienced practitioners can easily confuse anisotropic shadowing for real pathology such as a tendon tear.

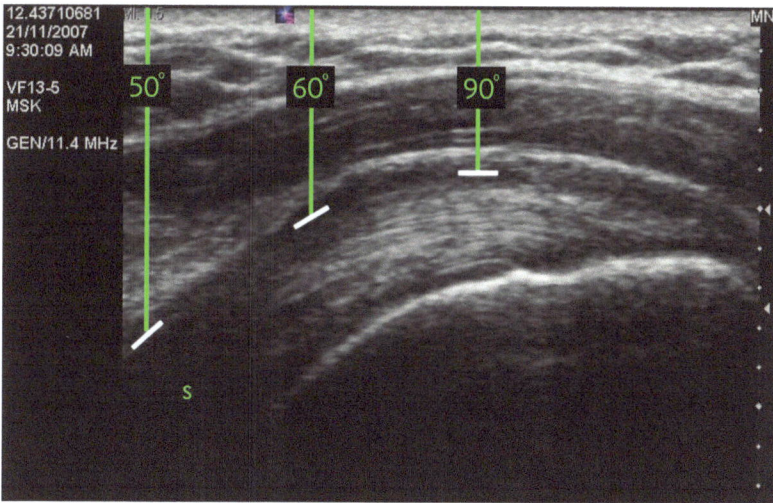

Figure 3.39: Normal supraspinatus tendon demonstrating good reflectivity and normal fibrillar structure in the region of normal (90°) incidence. As the tendon curves away from normal (60°, 50°), visualization of the tendon fibers is progressively lost in an enlarging zone of shadowing (s).

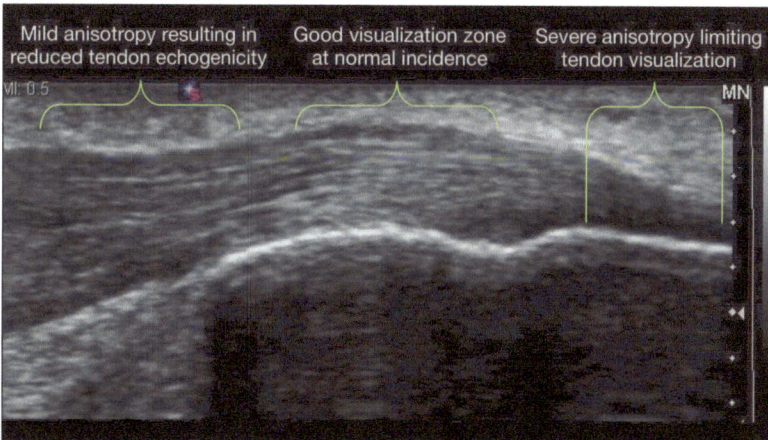

Figure 3.40: Normal Achilles tendon in longitudinal section demonstrating varying degrees of anisotropy with dropout at the tendon insertion.

Chapter 4

Beam Dimension Artifacts

The ultrasound beam is not infinitely thin. Instead it is a field of energy that has a defined pulse length (axial), width (beam-width) and depth (slice thickness). Reflectors are therefore not represented as discrete focal points. Instead they can be thought of as bricks or tiles. They are thin in the axial dimension, but are variably wide and variably deep.

4.1 Beamwidth artifact

Also known as

Beamwidth.

Causative mechanisms

The ultrasound beam is relatively wide. Lateral resolution is generally quite poor compared to axial resolution. This problem can easily be seen in ultrasound images because the image appears to be composed of fine horizontal lines, not of discrete square reflectors. Ultrasound reflectors are said to be non-isovolumetric, that is, they are not cuboidal in their dimensions. Instead, ultrasound reflectors can be likened to tiles. They are uniformly thin along the beam axis, variably wide (dependent on scan plane focusing) and variably deep (dependent on elevation focusing).

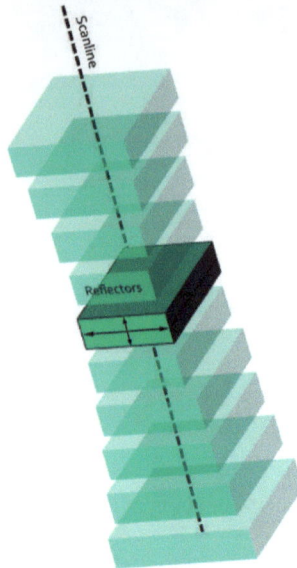

Figure 4.1: Each reflector appears in the image as an echo that has the form of a brick or tile, as shown here.

Which system assumptions have been breached?

The assumption that beam dimensions are small.

Typical appearance

Wide horizontal dimension of reflectors, lateral smearing, widening of lateral mass walls and organ boundaries, thickening of vessel walls when interrogated at angles other than normal incidence (90°). Beamwidth effects are particularly pronounced in the far-field when narrow apertures are used (focus is close to the transducer).

Can this artifact be reduced, eliminated or circumvented?

Beamwidth is a major problem in ultrasound imaging, especially when examining small structures. Small structures may prove difficult to resolve and/or there may be horizontal smearing of the structures making it difficult to determine their boundaries. Because spatial resolution is best along the beam axis (axial resolution), many standard ultrasound measurements are best performed along this beam dimension including: nuchal translucency, gallbladder wall thickness, bile duct diameter, intima-media thickness and aneurysm diameter measurement.

Ultrasound machines include a range of sophisticated technologies to assist with the reduction of beam width both in the pulse generation and echo reception components of beamforming. Some of these technologies are under direct control of the operator: transmit focusing, multiple focal zones, frequency selection, line density controls. Other technologies are built in and perform corrective actions in the background automatically: apodization, receive focusing, dynamic receive aperture.

There are a number of ways in which the operator can reduce beamwidth:

1   First and foremost, beamwidth is dependent on focusing. Adjusting the location of the transmit focus so that the structure of interest is in the focal zone of the beam will ensure the smallest beamwidth and therefore the best lateral resolution.

2   Multiple focal zones can be used to get large regions of the image into focus, however the trade off is a reduction in temporal resolution.

3   Increasing the transducer frequency on multifrequency capable systems or using a higher frequency transducer will reduce beamwidth because higher frequency beams are more directional.

4   Using a transducer of higher element density may be an option in centers where a range of different transducers is available.

5   Switching to tissue harmonic imaging also reduces beamwidth and slice thickness, but at the expense of frame rate.

6   Reduction of power output and gain may also help, but at the expense of sensitivity.

7   If the operator is using a conventional transducer and the object of interest lies in the near field, then the use of an acoustic standoff pad will increase the beam path and bring the object of interest into the elevation plane focus of the transducer. This can be helpful with small superficial structures, superficial musculoskeletal scanning and foreign bodies.

Is this artifact diagnostically useful?

No. Beamwidth artifact is never useful and the sonographer should always aim for the smallest beamwidth in the region of interest.

Beamwidth, an elusive image parameter

It is evident that beamwidth and the corresponding reflector size are highly variable. This can be nicely demonstrated using a simple experiment with a small reflector in a water bath, as shown in Figure 4.2. A 1mm thick metallic pin is being insonated using a high-frequency linear array transducer. The pin casts a prominent reverberation artifact.

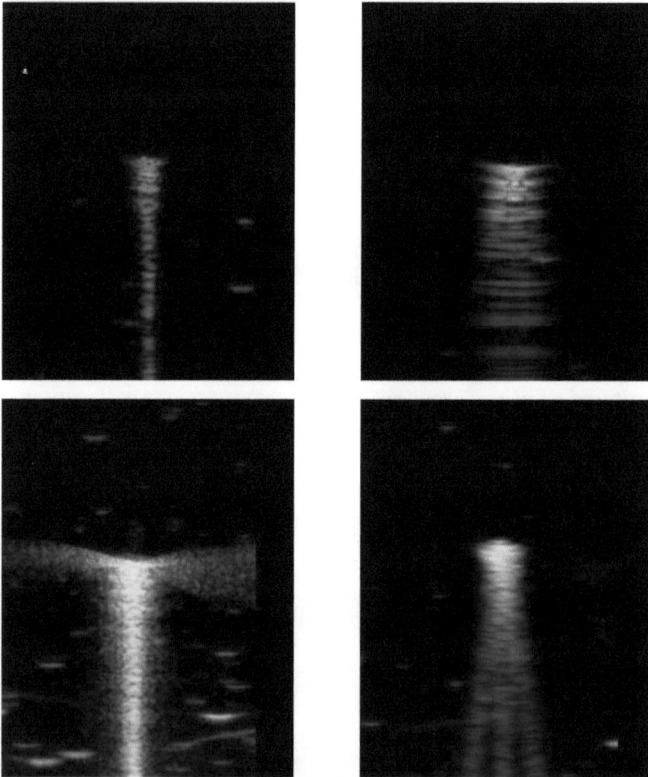

Figure 4.2: Top left: Focus at level of pin; optimal gain; no spatial compounding. Top right: Focus above level of pin; optimal gain; no spatial compounding. Bottom left: Focus above level of pin; high gain; no spatial compounding. Bottom right: Focus above level of pin; optimal gain; spatial compounding on.

In Figure 4.2 a variety of imaging parameters are being changed with dramatic effects on the apparent size (beamwidth) of the pin. The effects would be even more diverse if we used a variety of different transducers to repeat this experiment.

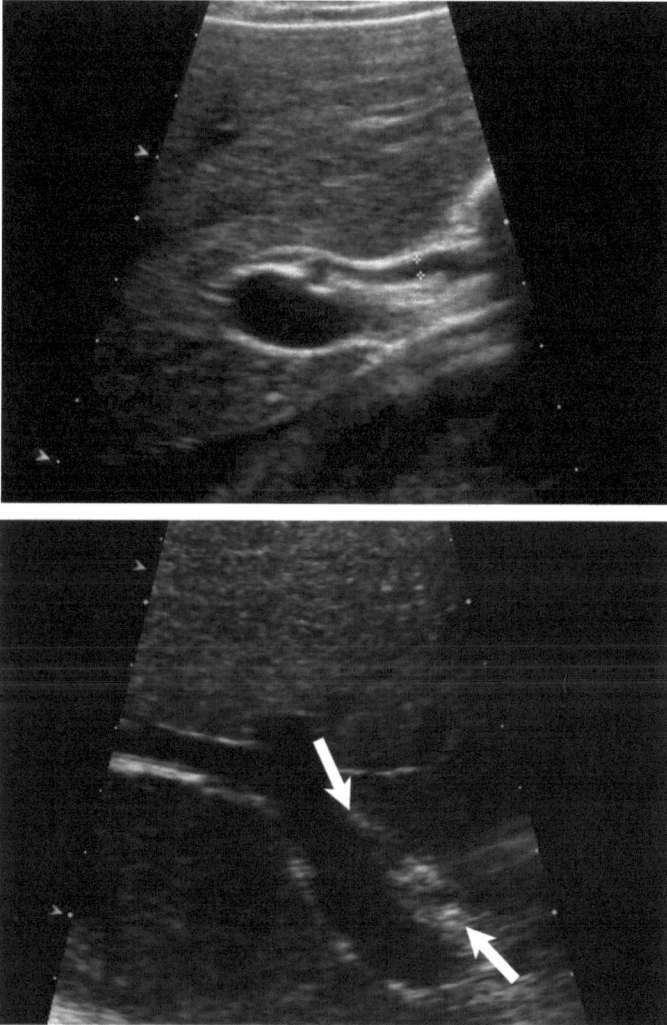

Figure 4.3: The bile duct is seen clearly when scanned at normal incidence (90°) in the upper image. When a different acoustic window is used and the bile duct is at an acute angle to the beam, it cannot be visualized because the beamwidth artifact fills the bile duct lumen (lower image). Arrows show the bile duct location.

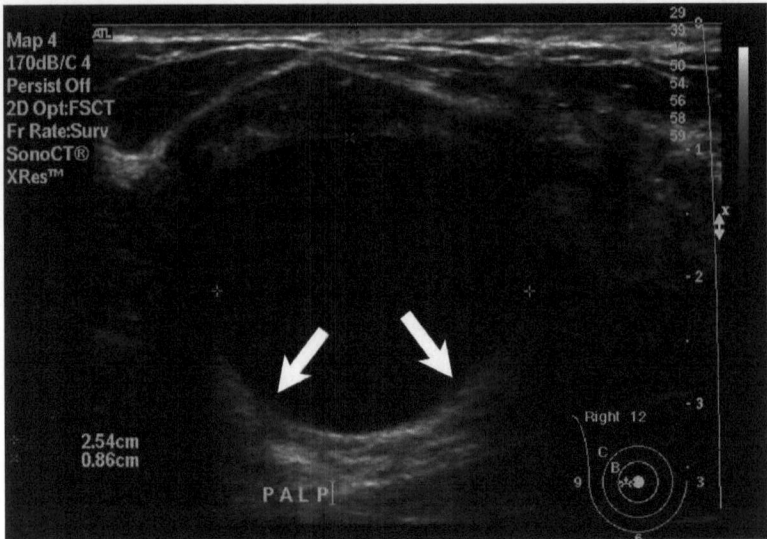

Figure 4.4: Simple cyst showing beamwidth artifact.

In Figure 4.4 the leading edge of the cyst is thin but the dependent wall of the cyst beyond the focal zone demonstrates beamwidth artifact (arrows). To reduce the beamwidth at the level of the artifact, the sonographer could lower the position of the focal zone but this would lead to a beamwidth problem in the leading edge of the cyst.

Alternatively, multiple focal zones could be used, but this would have a negative impact on frame rate. This may not be a problem in superficial imaging where the PRF is naturally high. But with deeper structures such as in abdominal imaging, the use of multiple focal zones may result in very low frame rates.

The beamwidth artifact is particularly pronounced with the use of small apertures, as shown in Figure 4.5. This occurs when the operator selects a shallow position of the dynamic transmit focus (indicated by the arrow) but maintains a deep field of view. Ultrasound pulses with narrow apertures suffer from wide angles of divergence resulting in progressively broader beamwidth. This can be seen in this image of a hemorrhagic ovarian cyst as increasingly larger reflector width along the scan line.

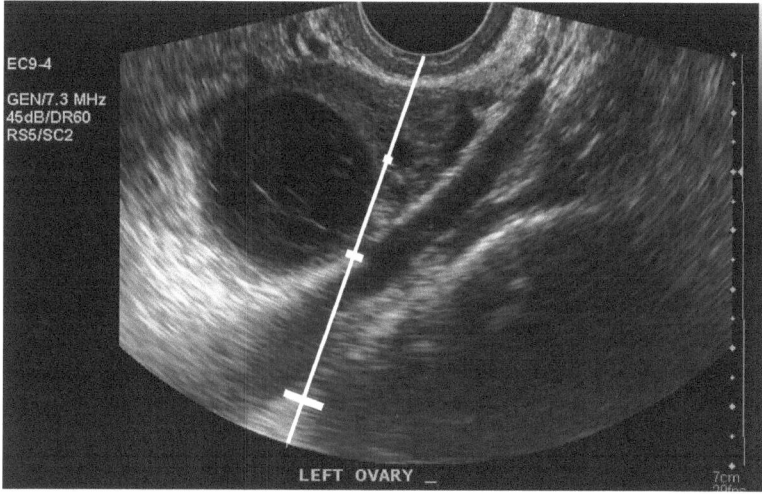

Figure 4.5: Image showing the impact of a shallow focus on beamwidth artifact.

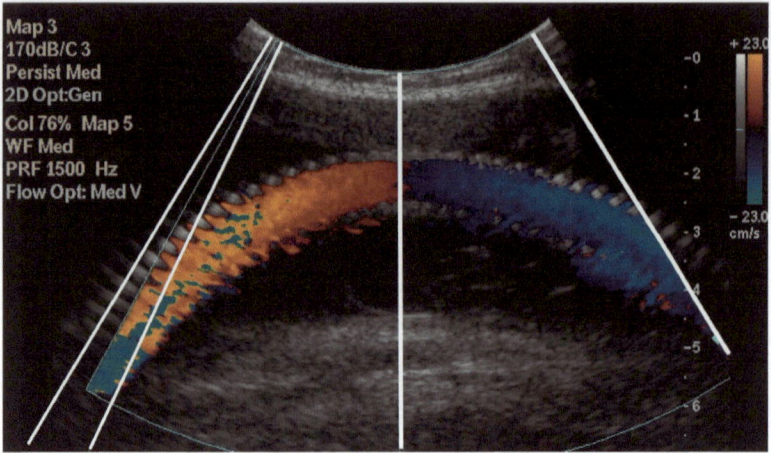

Figure 4.6: Beamwidth artifact is responsible for the apparent variation of thickness of this synthetic arterial bypass graft. Note that the most favorable scanning approach where beam dimensions are the smallest is at 90° to the graft. This approach takes advantage of high axial resolution which is always far superior to lateral resolution.

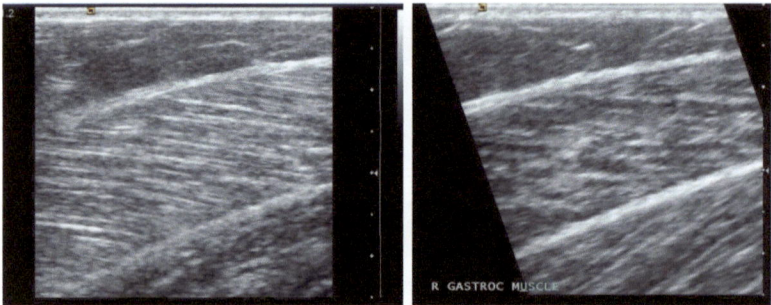

Figure 4.8: These images show the same medial gastrocnemius muscle scanned with two different beam-steering approaches. Note how much finer the fibrillar pattern of the muscle appears when imaged at 90° incidence (left) when compared to the beam-steered image on the right. The tissue reflectors appear much thicker in the right image, largely due to unfavorable beamwidth.

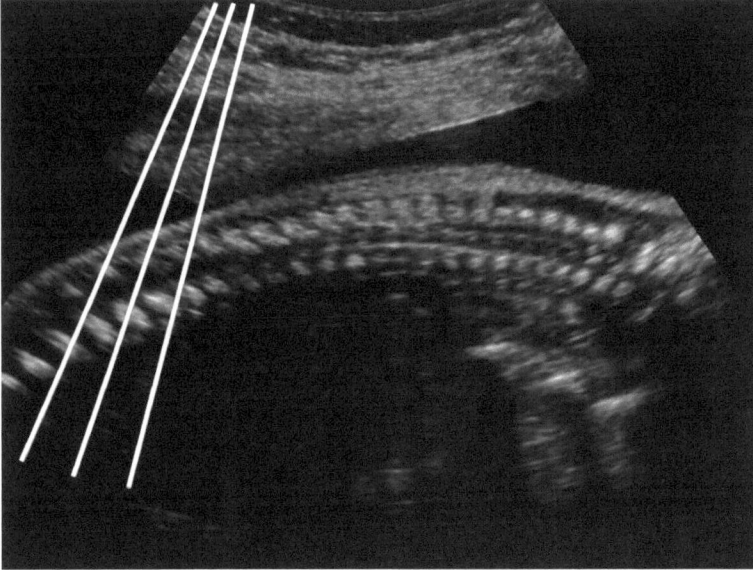

Figure 4.7: In this image of the fetal spine, the beamwidth artifact in the left side of the image causes the vertebral bodies to appear enlarged. The beamwidth problem is accentuated in this part of the image due to multiple factors: 1) unfavorable (acute) angle of incidence, 2) the position of the reflectors in the far-zone (beyond the focal point) and 3) loss of lateral resolution due to the divergent nature of the scanlines when a curvilinear transducer is used.

Beamwidth and beam thickness (slice thickness) affect the appearance of a range of other artifacts. For example the tendency of a highly reflecting/attenuating structure to shadow is heavily influenced by beamwidth. If the beamwidth is larger than the structure, shadowing may not occur.

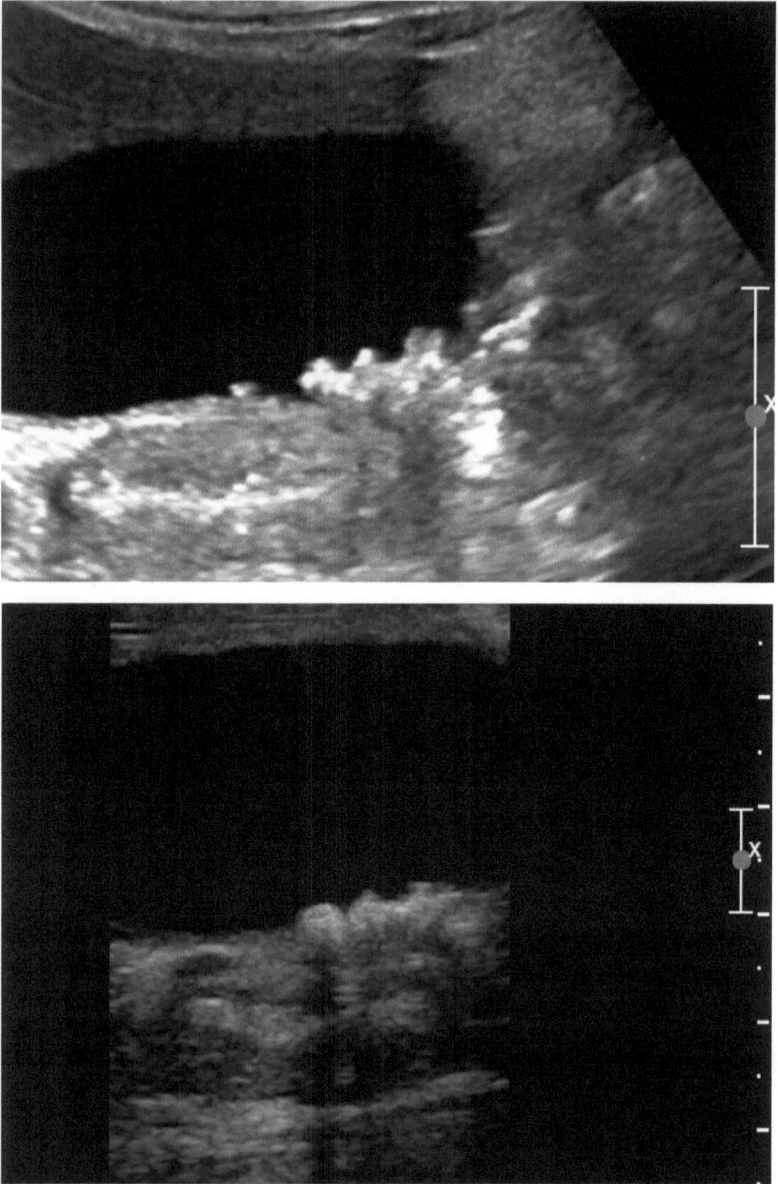

Figure 4.9: In this example, the gallstones within the gallbladder do not shadow when a low frequency transducer is used (upper image). Higher frequency transducers have narrower, more directional beams and greater line density. Shadowing of the gallstones is clearly demonstrated (lower image).

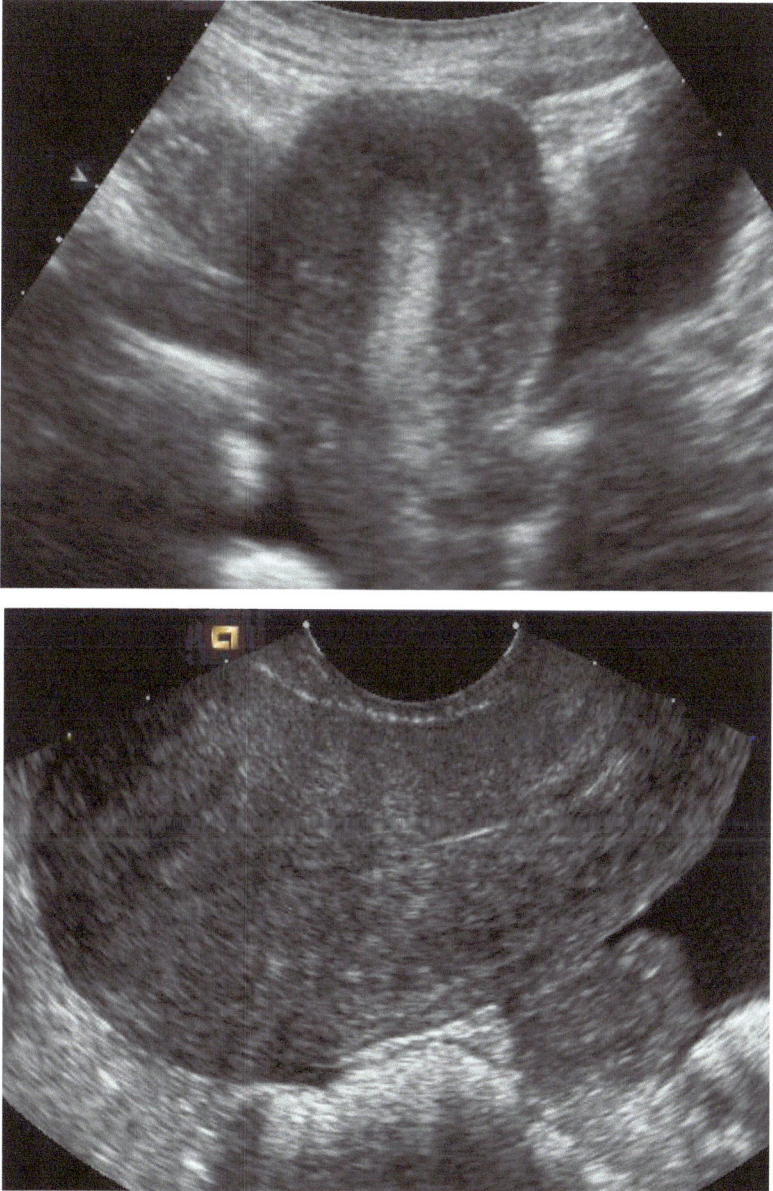

Figure 4.10: Beam-width artifact resulting in thickened secretory endometrial appearance on transabdominal scan (upper image) in a patient with normal early proliferative endometrium on transvaginal scan (lower image). Note that better scanning approach (normal incidence) is achieved transvaginally because the scanning approach is along the axial beam dimension.

Clinical limitations of beam dimensions

Beam dimensions are the determinants of spatial image resolution. It is often possible to improve spatial resolution and in turn contrast resolution by applying the simple principle of using the highest frequency transducer as long as penetration is adequate.

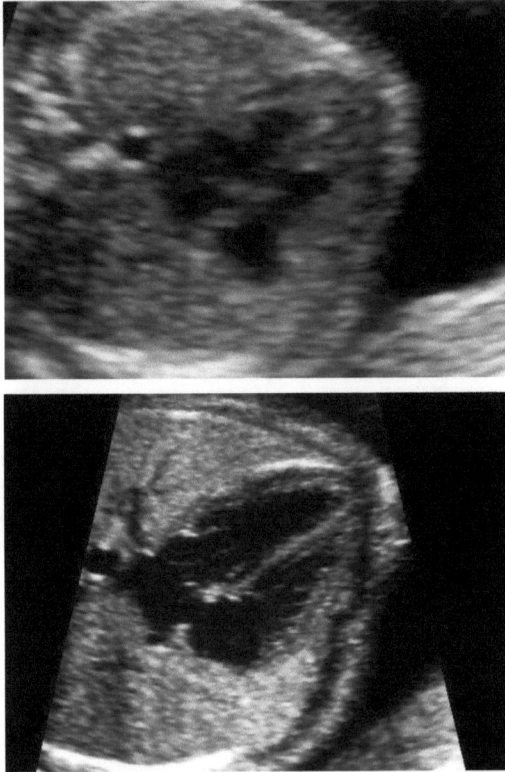

Figure 4.11: In this example fetal cardiac survey is being performed at 19 weeks gestational age. The upper image is obtained using a 4-1MHz transducer. The image suffers from poor axial resolution, poor lateral resolution and poor slice thickness which negatively impacts on contrast resolution. The image is diagnostically inadequate and suggests the presence of a ventricular septal defect (VSD). Marked improvement in image quality was achieved when the operator switched to 9-4MHz transducer (lower image) revealing a normal heart. The importance of using the highest frequency transducer possible cannot be overemphasized. Unfortunately this fundamental rule is sometimes ignored by ultrasound operators.

Clinical limitations of beam dimensions on 3D ultrasound

The influence of beam dimensions on the visualization of small objects can also be demonstrated in 3D ultrasound.

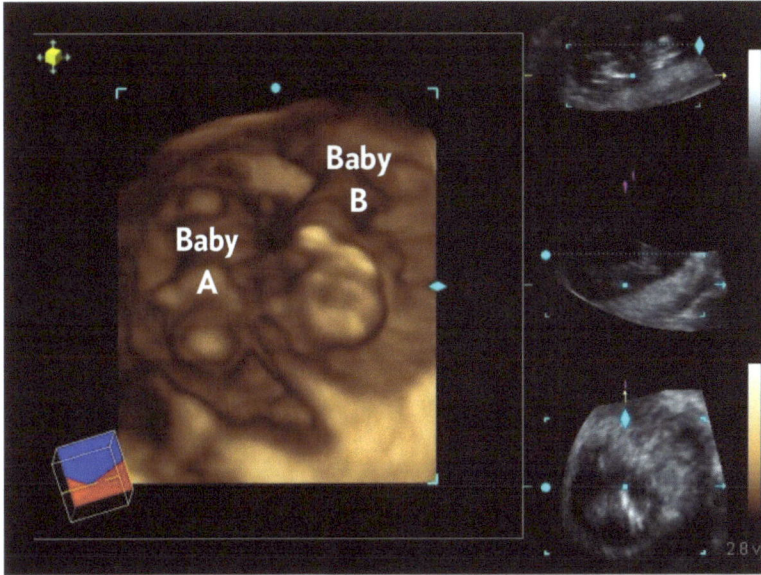

Figure 4.12: In this image, a 10 week dichorionic twin gestation was scanned using a 1-5MHz mechanical 3D transducer. The two fetuses are barely recognizable and fine body detail is not discernible. Sonographers sometimes describe this effect as 'plasticine' or 'jellybean' appearance. It is due to the large beam dimensions in the axial, lateral and slice thickness planes compared with the small dimensions of the fetal parts.

The effect of unfavorable beam dimensions and the non-isovolumetric nature of ultrasound voxels can also be seen in 3D ultrasound at later gestational ages.

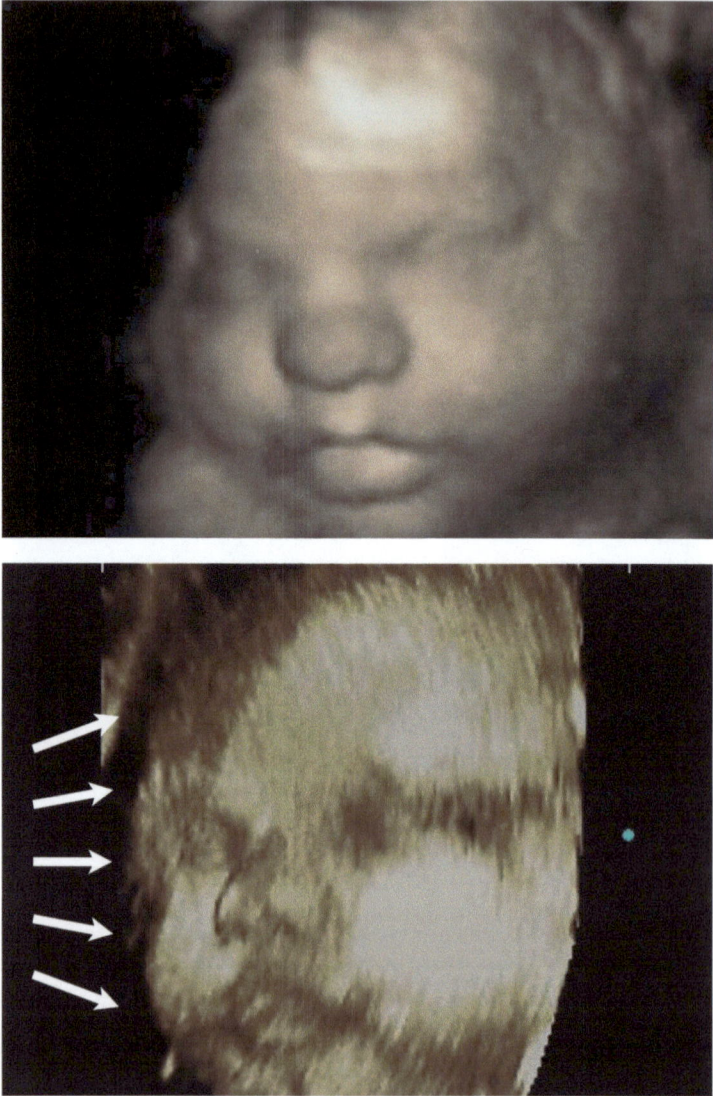

Figure 4.13: Both of the fetuses shown here were imaged at 28 weeks. The upper image was acquired at a favorable angle with the baby facing in the direction of the transducer. The image is clear, detailed and the voxel widths and heights are uniform across the image. The lower image was acquired with the baby on its side and facing slightly away. The direction of the incident beams is shown (arrows). Following acquisition, the image was rotated to a portrait format. The image appears streaky because the non-axial approach results in variable beamwidth with depth.

4.2 Slice thickness

Also known as

Partial volume effect.

Causative mechanisms

The ultrasound beam is relatively wide in the thickness plane. Slice thickness is usually at least as poor as lateral resolution and often worse. This means that the operator is not visualizing a thin plane of anatomy on the 2D image but rather a thick slab of information which is all averaged together into the visible section. Large slice thickness is undesirable as it reduces contrast resolution and creates uncertainty about the precise location of small objects. In order to reduce slice thickness, most transducers in use today contain an acoustic lens which runs along the length of the array. The slice thickness focus is therefore fixed by lens characteristics and cannot be altered by the operator. The exception to this is 1½D array transducers or matrix array transducers which can dynamically focus the beam in both scan plane and the elevation plane.

Which system assumptions have been breached?

The assumption that beam dimensions are small.

Typical appearance

Echoes from behind or in front of the expected sectional plane are contaminating the image. For example, a small anechoic object (cyst, vessel) may fill in with echoes from in front and behind the central plane of section. Large anechoic objects (such as the gallbladder or urinary bladder) may contain low-level echoes attributable to bowel gas behind the plane of section.

Can this artifact be reduced, eliminated or circumvented?

There are a number of ways that slice thickness can be reduced:

1 Increasing the transducer frequency or using a higher frequency transducer will reduce slice thickness because higher frequency beams are more directional.

2   Switching to tissue harmonic imaging also reduces beamwidth
     and slice thickness, but at the expense of frame rate.

3   Reduction of power output and gain may also help, but at the
     expense of sensitivity.

4   If the operator is using a conventional transducer and the object
     of interest lies in the near field, then the use of an acoustic
     standoff pad can help elongate the beam path and bring the object
     of interest into the elevation plane focus of the transducer. This
     can be helpful with small superficial structures, superficial
     musculoskeletal scanning and foreign bodies.

Is this artifact diagnostically useful?

The slice thickness artifact is always undesirable in 2D imaging. In 3D
ultrasound imaging, however, there are several circumstances in which
large slice thickness can be useful; this special technique is referred to as
"thick-slice" volume rendering.

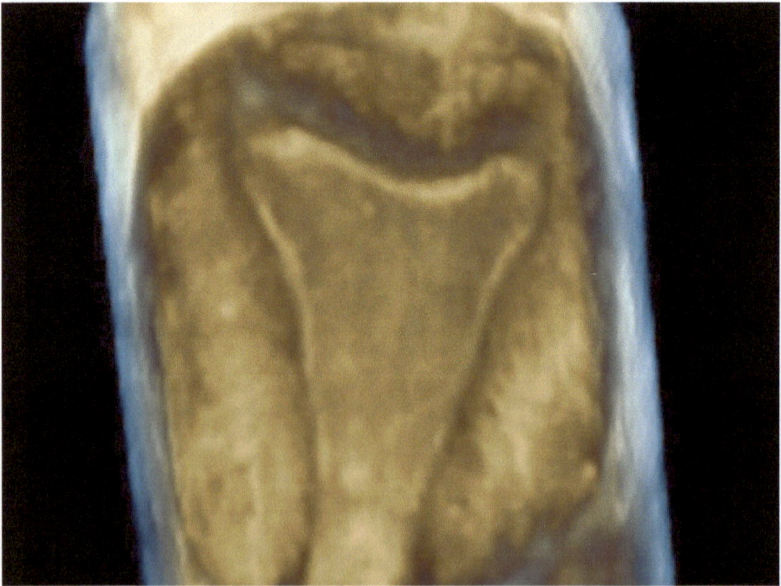

Figure 4.14: Thick-slice volume rendering of the uterus and endometrium.

The idea behind thick-slice rendering is that averaging multiple 2D slices into a single view can result in smoother image texture and accentuate subtle findings because a subtle finding will have an additive effect over several image slices.

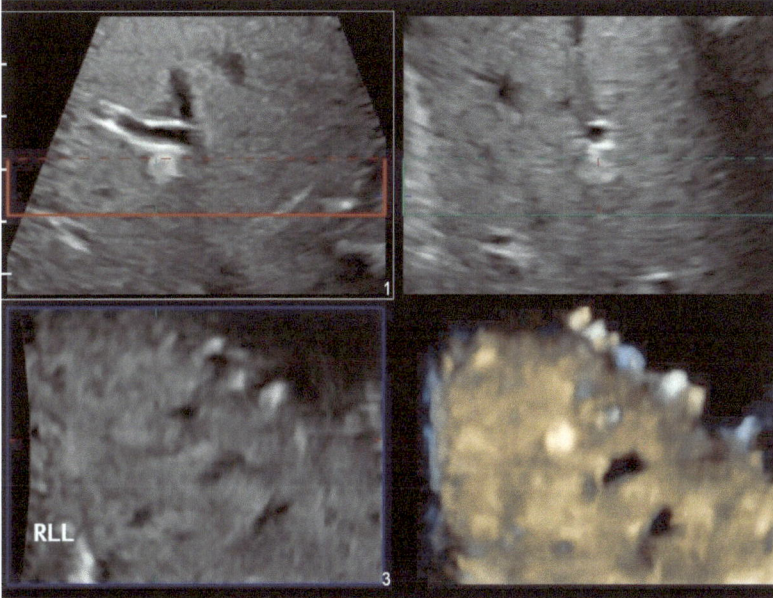

Figure 4.15: 3D multiplanar reformats (3D MPR) and thick-slice volume rendering of a tiny hemangioma. Note the improved lesion conspicuity in the thick-slice image (bottom right).

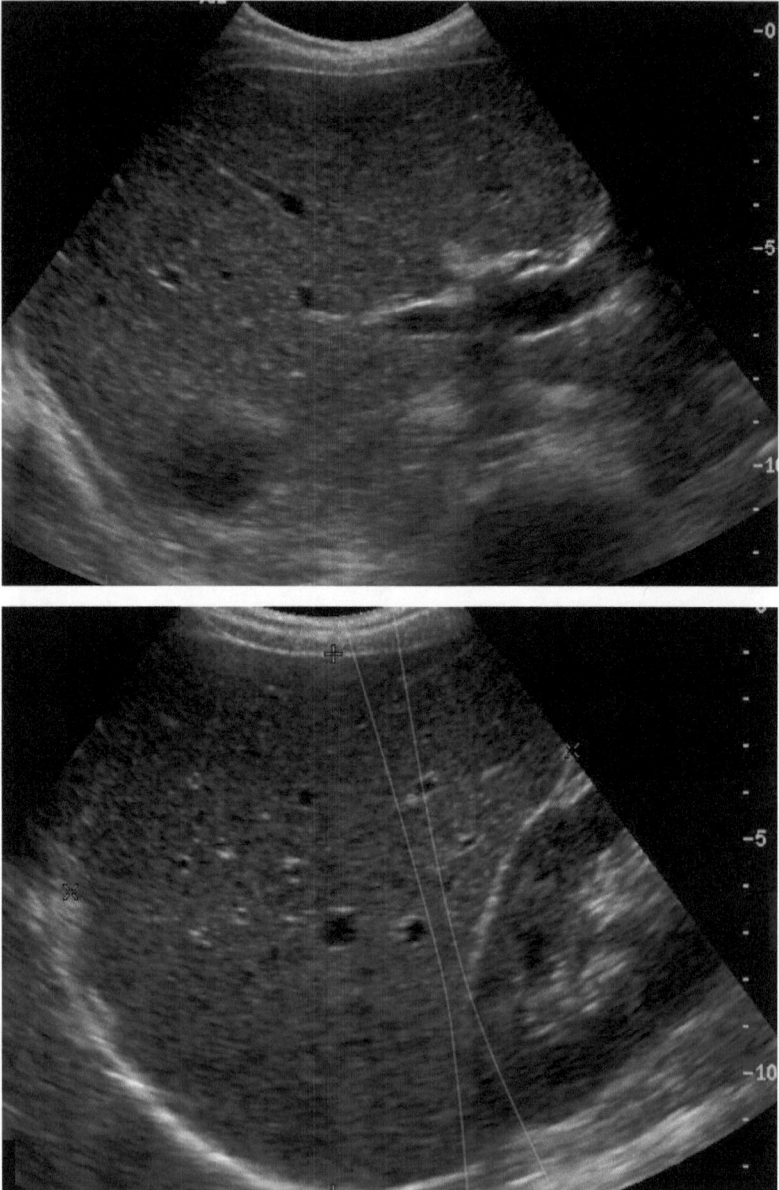

Figure 4.16: In this example the sonographer obtained a transverse section of the liver (upper image) and captured the upper pole of the kidney in the same slice effectively creating the appearance of a liver mass (pseudo-mass). Longitudinal view of the same region (lower image) shows the normal liver without any masses. The problematic slice-thickness region is shown in the lower image.

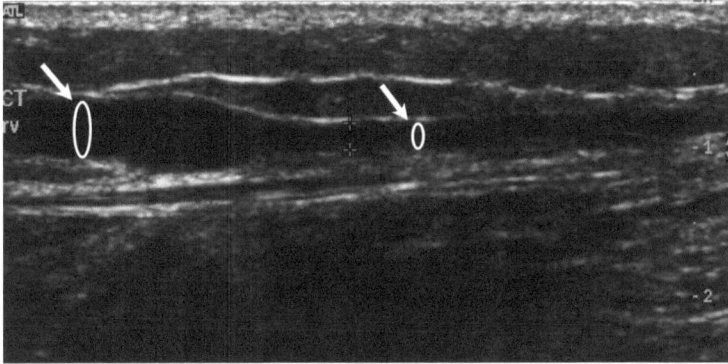

Figure 4.17: This patent lower extremity vein reduces in diameter from left to right. In the left part of the image, the diameter of the vessel is larger than the slice thickness and the vessel is anechoic. In the right part of the image, the vessel diameter is smaller than the slice thickness and echoes from behind and in front of the vessel contaminate the lumen. Apart from attempting to reduce slice thickness, the sonographer can use color Doppler or transverse compression sonography to ensure the vessel is not thrombosed.

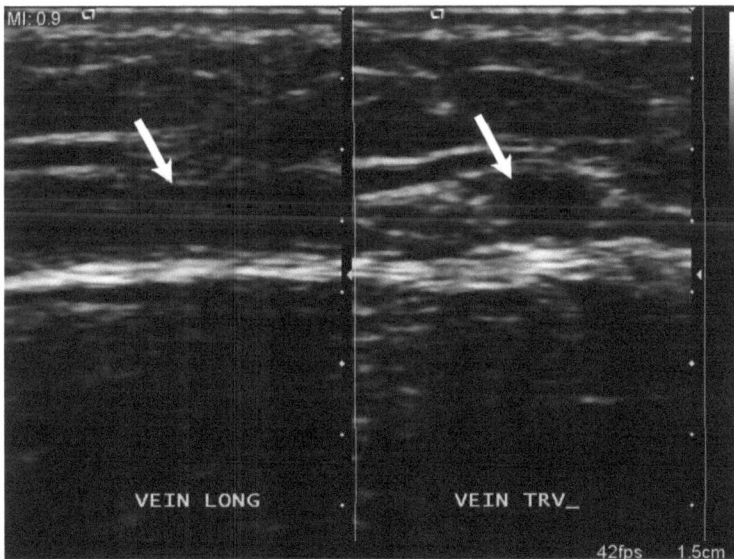

Figure 4.18: A small vessel is shown in dual-screen in longitudinal section (left) and transverse section (right). The vessel size is smaller than the slice thickness and the vessel lumen in the longitudinal section is contaminated by echoes from behind and in-front of the lumen. This problem does not occur in the transverse section where the vein is clearly visualized and appears anechoic.

When using conventional array transducers (linear array, curvilinear array), it is useful to remember that axial resolution is always better than lateral resolution and lateral resolution is usually better than slice thickness.

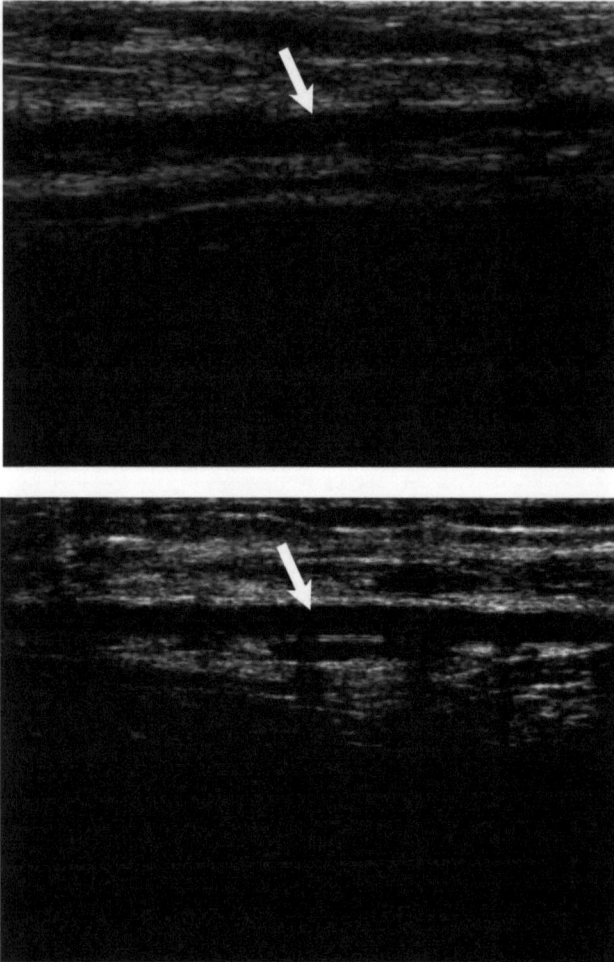

Figure 4.19: A small vessel (radial artery) is being interrogated using a 9-4MHz linear array transducer operating in fundamental mode at 9MHz (upper image). The same vessel is then interrogated using a 5-17MHz linear array transducer operating in harmonic mode at 14MHz (lower image). The vessel in the upper image is echo-filled due to the large slice thickness of this transducer. A much higher resolution image and the normal anechoic nature of the vessel is revealed when the operator switches to a higher frequency and uses harmonic imaging.

4.3 Sidelobe artifacts

Causative mechanisms

The ultrasound beam comprises a main lobe of acoustic energy centrally with other weaker lobes surrounding the main lobe in all directions. The generation of sidelobes is an unfortunate and unavoidable byproduct of acoustics and is fundamentally linked to the Huygen's principle. Ultrasound is generated by the vibration of piezoelectric elements. The elements act as if they are composed of a large number of tiny sources of sound. The ultrasound beam (main energy lobe) is a region of constructive interference between the wavelets of sound from all the point sources. Sidelobes represent other regions of constructive interference outside the main lobe (see diagram overleaf). The main lobe and side lobes are in turn separated by regions of destructive interference.

Which system assumptions have been breached?

The assumption that echoes only originate from the central axis of the beam.

Typical appearance

Wide horizontal smear of echogenicity in an anechoic or hypoechoic structure which seems to emanate from a highly echogenic structure. Sidelobe artifacts are particularly easy to appreciate where fluid structures (such as bladder, gallbladder, vessels, amniotic cavity) are in close proximity to a markedly echogenic structure (bowel gas, bone, stones). Because sidelobes are three dimensional, it is possible to visualize the artifacts in a section that does not show the original object.

Common misconceptions

Students of ultrasound often confuse sidelobe artifacts with beamwidth artifact. Sidelobe artifacts are usually far greater in span than beamwidth artifacts, often affecting large segments of the field of view and sometimes the entire field of view.

Can this artifact be reduced, eliminated or circumvented?

Ultrasound machines try to limit the impact of sidelobes through various built-in technologies such as apodization and receive focusing. The operator has no control over these features. The operator can try to reduce the impact of sidelobes by using tissue harmonic imaging. Reduction of acoustic output power and gain can also reduce the appearance of the artifact, but at the expense of sensitivity.

Is this artifact diagnostically useful?

No. This artifact is a nuisance and is never useful.

The generation of the main lobe and sidelobes

As shown in Figure 4.20, small wavelets of sound originating at the transducer surface begin to combine through the effects of constructive interference to form a central peak acoustic energy zone known as the ultrasound beam or main lobe. Other weaker off-axis regions of constructive interference also occur and these are known as sidelobes.

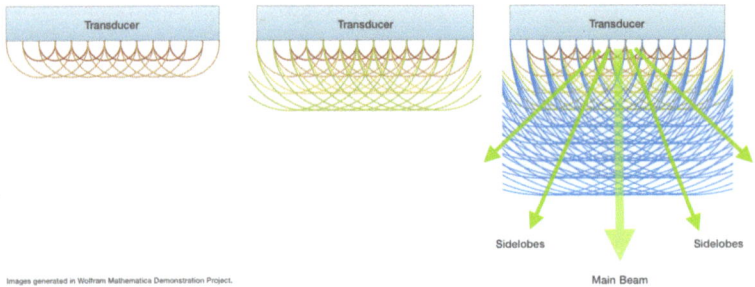

Figure 4.20: Diagram showing how sidelobes are generated.

Sidelobe artifact

Sidelobes are best appreciated in anechoic structures.

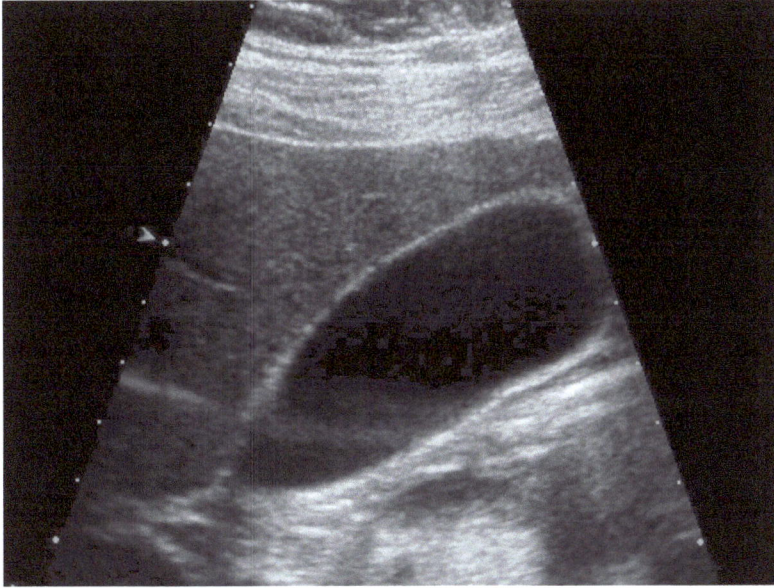

Figure 4.21: In this image, a sidelobe artifact is seen projected into the gallbladder and liver.

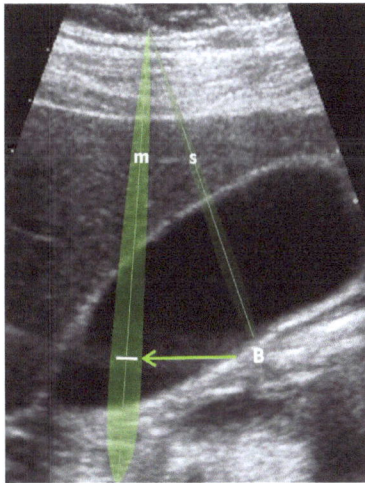

Figure 4.22: The generation of the artifact in Figure 4.21 is shown here. The main beam (m) is interrogating the anechoic gallbladder lumen. A sidelobe (s) of the beam encounters highly echogenic bowel gas (B). These echoes will return along the sidelobe back to the transducer. The echoes will be assumed to originate from the central axis of the beam (m) and will be projected along the beam path.

The negative effect of the sidelobe artifact on the image can sometimes be dramatically reduced by using a different angle of approach (see Figure 4.23).

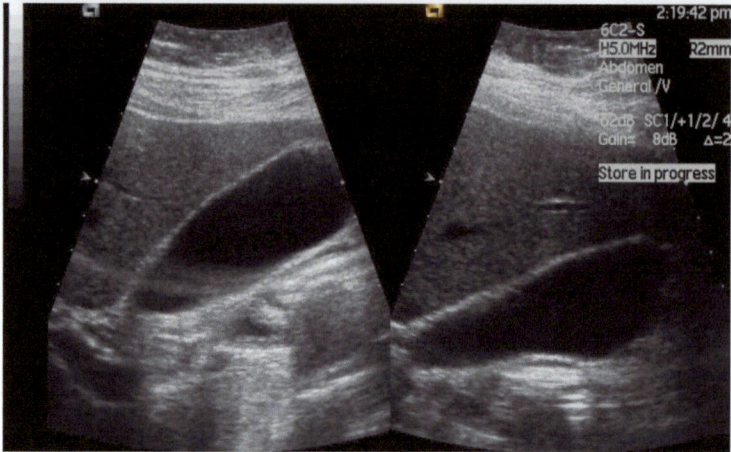

Figure 4.23: A prominent sidelobe artifact is seen in the image on the left. Changing the angle of approach so that the sidelobe artifact is now projected below the level of the gallbladder results in an improved image.

Sidelobe artifacts are common in obstetric imaging where two factors favor their existence: 1) large anechoic regions of amniotic fluid, 2) highly echogenic structures (bones) in close proximity to fluid. Two examples are shown in Figures 4.24 and 4.25.

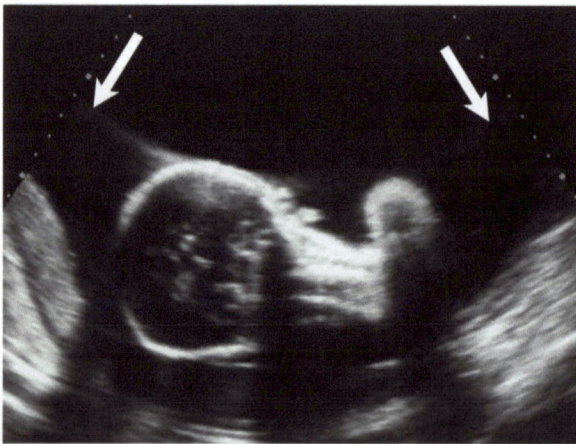

Figure 4.24: Sidelobe artifacts associated with the fetal skull in a mid-trimester fetus scanned transabdominally.

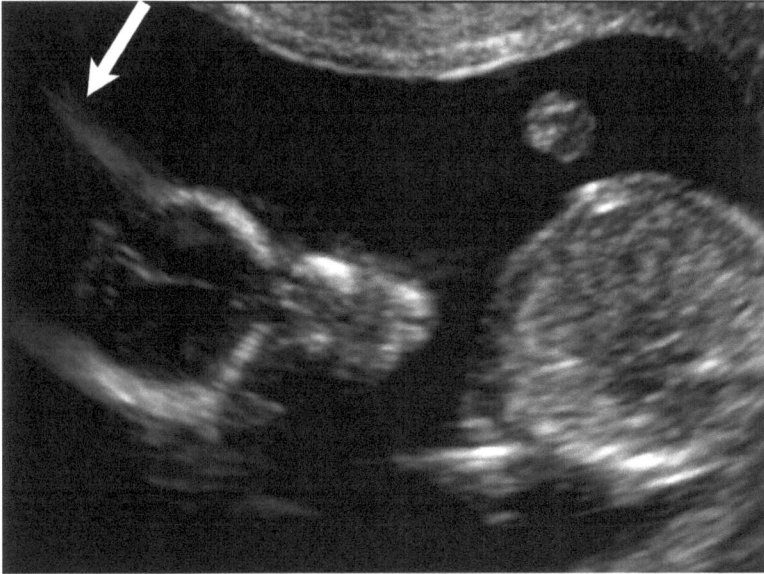

Figure 4.25: Sidelobe artifact in a 12-week fetus scanned transvaginally.

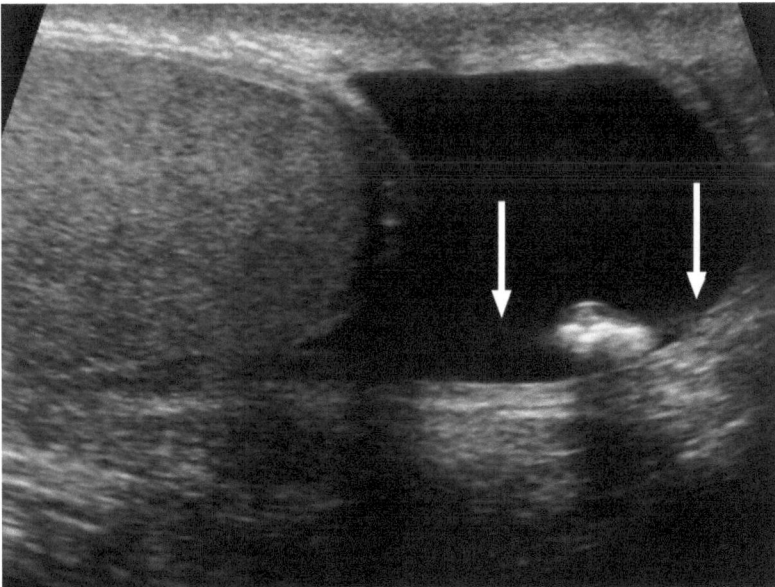

Figure 4.26: A sidelobe artifact associated with a scrotal pearl within a mild hydrocele.

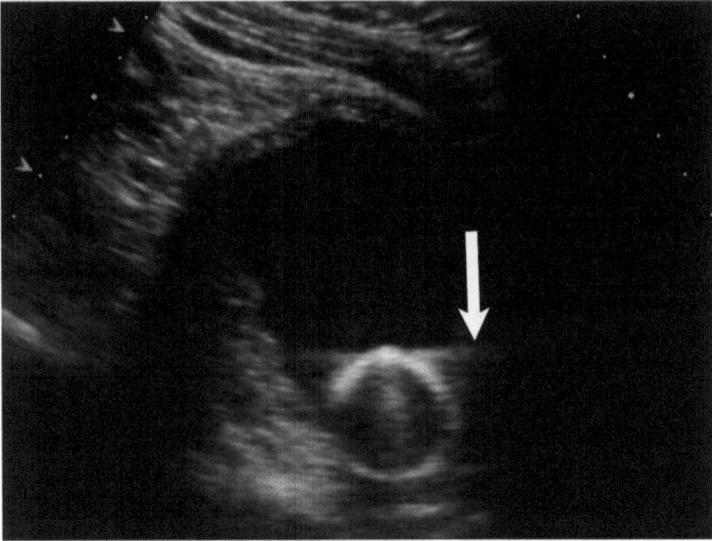

Figure 4.27: A sidelobe artifact generated by a Foley Catheter is seen in the mid-sagittal section of the bladder.

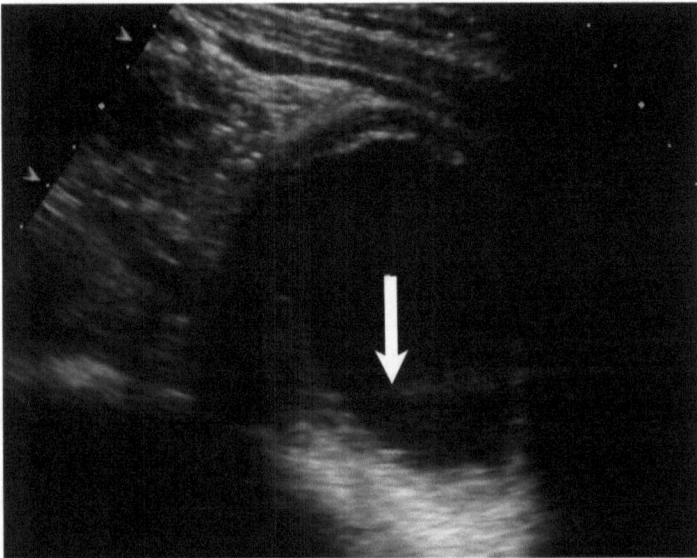

Figure 4.28: In the left or right parasagittal section, the sidelobe artifact caused by the catheter is still visualized (arrow) even though the causative object is not present in the same plane of section. This occurs because sidelobes not only exist in the plane of imaging but also in the elevation plane.

Chapter 5

Refraction

Refraction is the change of beam direction that occurs when an ultrasound beam encounters a boundary between two acoustic regions with different propagation speeds. The angle of incidence must be non-perpendicular for refraction to occur. Refraction contributes to several artifacts already discussed in this book including edge shadowing and anisotropic shadowing. Unique refraction scenarios occur in the abdomen due to the symmetrical refracting nature of the rectus abdominis muscles which behave like a pair of acoustic lenses. Apparent widening, bending, duplication or triplication of structures may occur in the ultrasound image.

5.1 Refraction ghost artifacts

Also known as

Duplication, ghost artifact

Causative mechanisms

In a transverse view of the abdomen, the rectus abdominis muscles act as two acoustic lenses and refract the ultrasound beam. Usually, the refraction effect is towards the midline. Because the machine assumes a straight beam path, an object which lies in the midline may be projected laterally which results in widening, duplication or triplication of this object.

Which system assumptions have been breached?

The assumption that the speed of sound is constant and the assumption that the beam and echoes travel along a straight path.

Typical appearance

Apparent widening, bending, side-by-side duplication or side-by-side triplication of abdominal or pelvic structures when imaged in the midline in transverse section. The most classic appearance involves apparent duplication of the SMA or duplication of a single gestational sac resulting in the appearance of twin sacs. The artifact disappears if the operator moves the transducer laterally away from the midline.

Common misconceptions

Students of ultrasound often assume that artifactual duplication of an object is always caused by the mirror image artifact. Refraction can cause duplication or triplication of an object. In the case of refraction, the false objects are always located laterally to the original object whereas in case of mirror image the false object is always located behind the acoustic mirror.

Can this artifact be reduced, eliminated or circumvented?

This artifact can be eliminated by sliding the transducer laterally so that it is not resting over both rectus abdominis muscles.

Is this artifact diagnostically useful?

No. This artifact can lead to confusing anatomical appearances and is never useful.

Refraction ghost artifact

An optical analogy of the ghost artifact can be demonstrated using two round glasses and a small object, in this case a tomato. Depending on the viewing angle (and other physical parameters), one can demonstrate a range of interesting refraction effects.

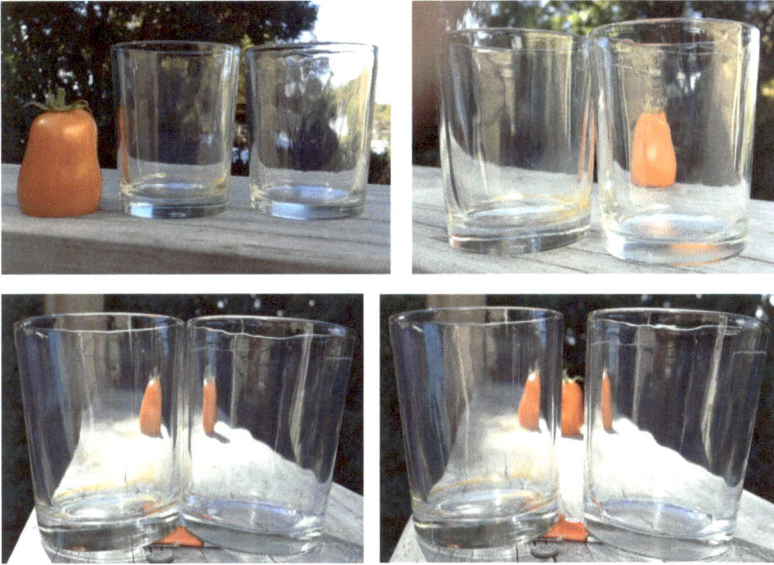

Figure 5.1: When the line of sight is directed through one glass only, only one tomato is seen (top right). If the line of sight is directed through the two closely adjacent glasses, the following effects can be seen: duplication (bottom left), triplication (bottom right).

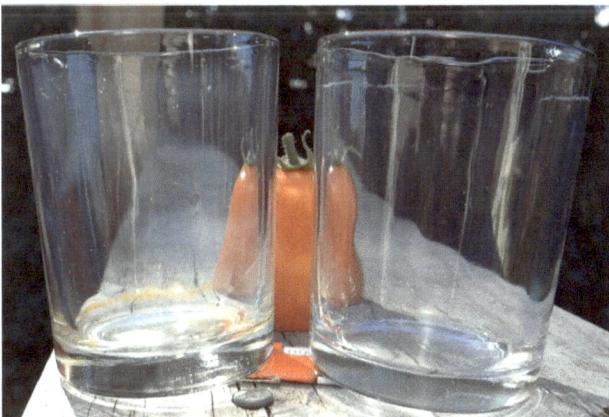

Figure 5.2: Refraction can also cause distortion and widening of objects in the image.

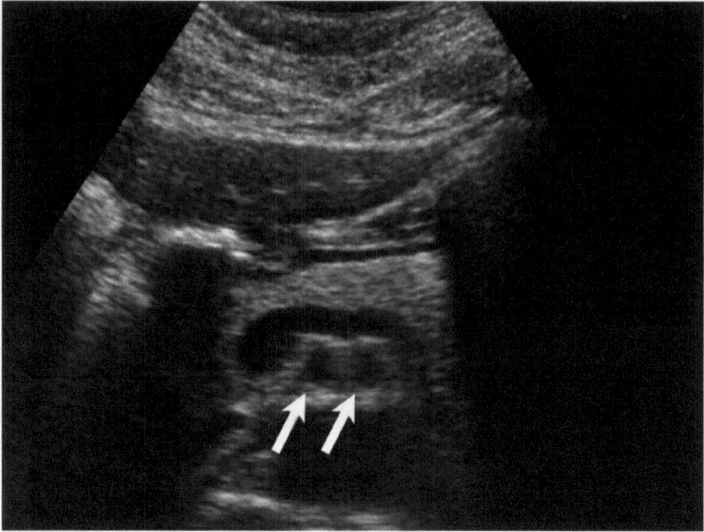

Figure 5.3: The superior mesenteric artery (SMA) appears duplicated in this image. The image is ambiguous. It could represent true anatomical variants which often occur at this location (such as the common hepatic artery branching off the SMA instead of the celiac axis) or the image could represent a refraction artifact.

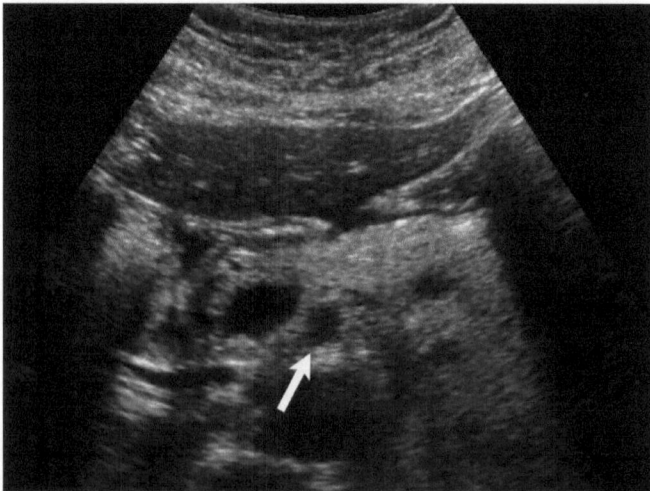

Figure 5.4: This is the same patient as shown in Figure 5.3. Moving the transducer laterally has caused the artifact to disappear, confirming the artifactual nature of the second vessel.

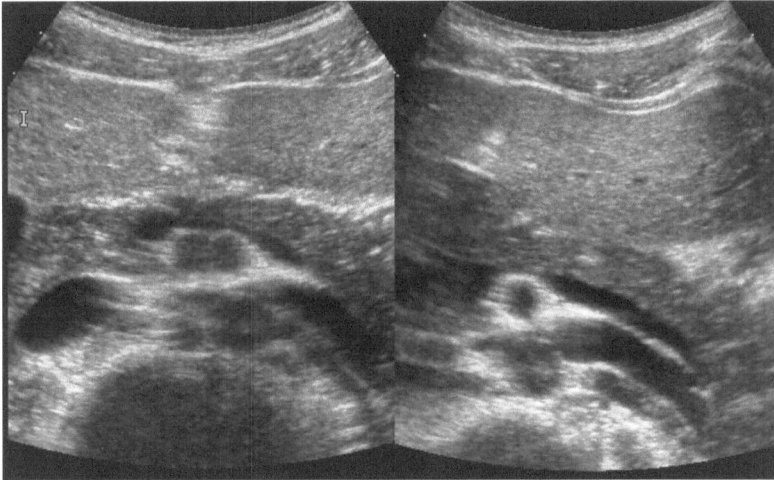

Figure 5.5: Another nice example of apparent duplication of the SMA (left frame).

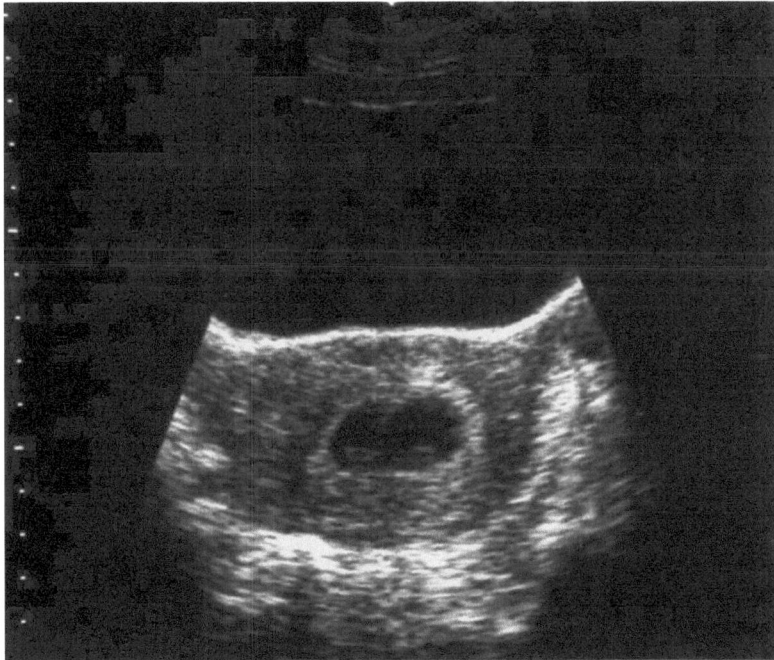

Figure 5.6: In this image the refraction artifact gives the impression of a twin pregnancy by duplicating a single gestational sac.

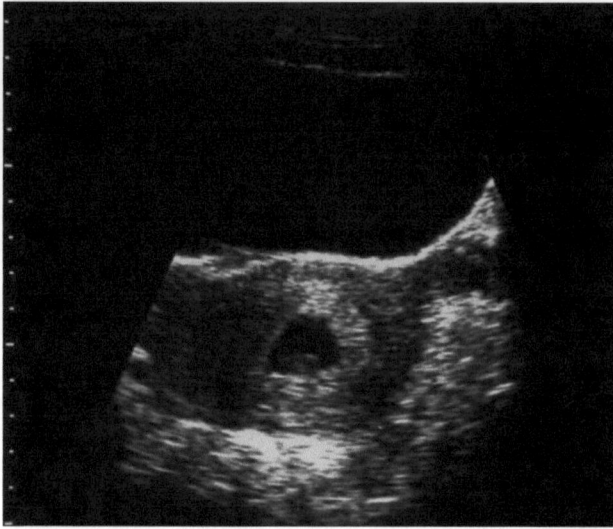

Figure 5.7: *The same patient as shown in the previous figure. The probe has been moved and the apparent duplication has disappeared.(Images courtesy Roger Gent, Adelaide. Reproduced by permission.)*

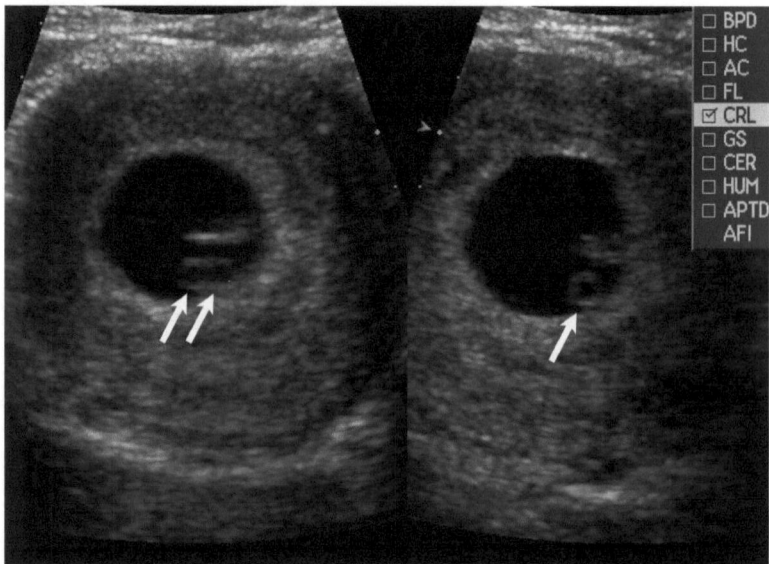

Figure 5.8: *The refraction artifact causes duplication of the yolk sac (left image) giving the impression of a monochorionic twin pregnancy. Repositioning of the transducer yields an improved view showing a solitary yolk sac.*

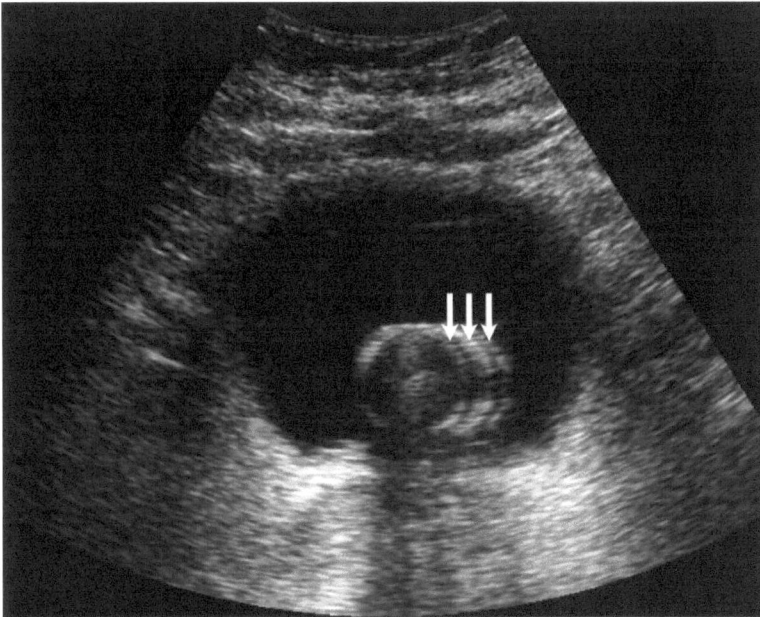

Figure 5.9: Partial ghosting of a Foley catheter with 3 copies of the left lateral catheter wall.

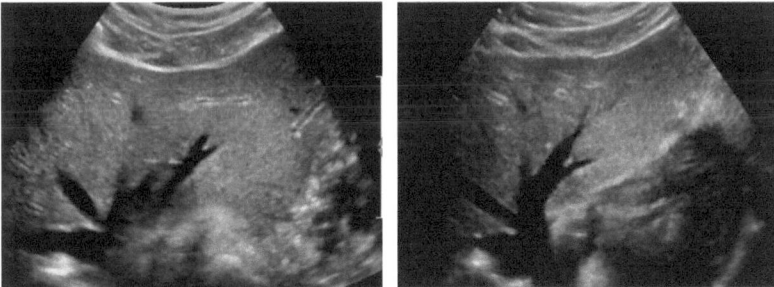

Figure 5.10: Duplication of the left hepatic vein branches is seen in the left image. Repositioning of the transducer laterally eliminates the artifact (right).

Not a refraction ghost

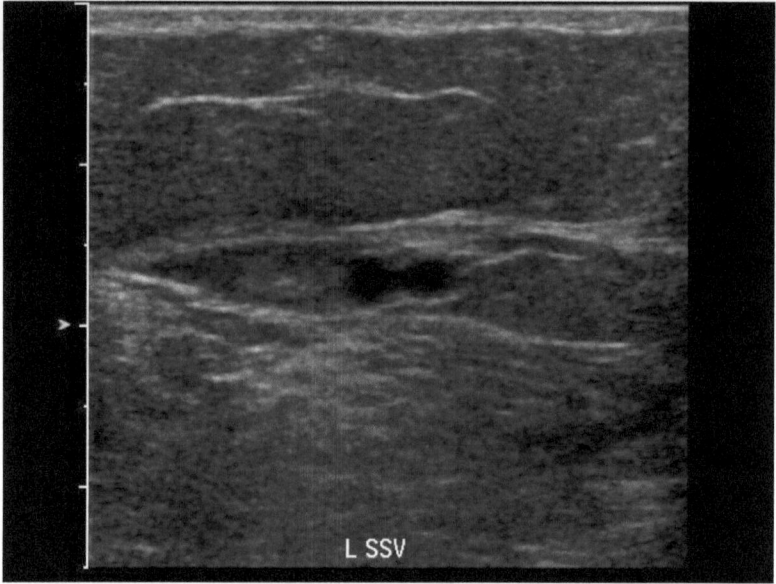

Figure 5.11: Refraction ghosting usually only occurs in the abdomen and is due to the double lens effect of the two rectus abdominis muscles. There is no other anatomical region prone to this type of refraction. This image shows true anatomical duplication of the small saphenous vein.

5.2 Refraction: distortion and defocusing

Causative mechanisms

The bending of an ultrasound beam due to refraction can lead to distortion and defocusing of parts of the image. For instance, if a large anatomical structure spans parts of the image that are not affected by refraction as well as parts of the image that are affected by refraction, the structure may appear distorted.

Which system assumptions have been breached?

The assumption that the speed of sound is constant and the assumption that the beam and echoes travel along a straight path.

Typical appearance

The appearance is variable, but in general the image appears distorted, blurred or defocused.

Can this artifact be reduced, eliminated or circumvented?

Refraction artifacts can be successfully eliminated by using different acoustic window. Often a very slight change in transducer position and angulation can eliminate the artifact.

Is this artifact diagnostically useful?

No. This artifact is never useful.

Refraction - distortion and defocusing

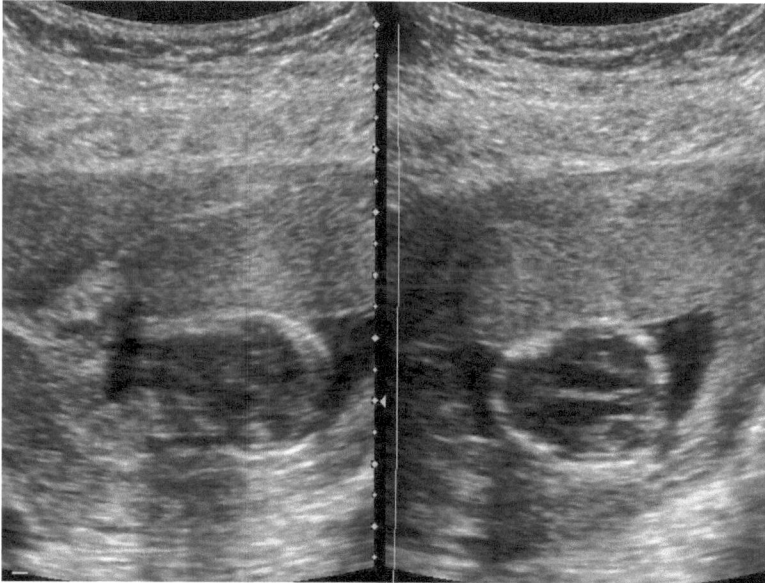

Figure 5.12: Dual image showing the same 12 week fetal head. Refraction defocusing is apparent in the left image with partial refraction ghosting of the anterior skull edge. A slight lateral change in transducer position resulted in the improved diagnostic image on the right.

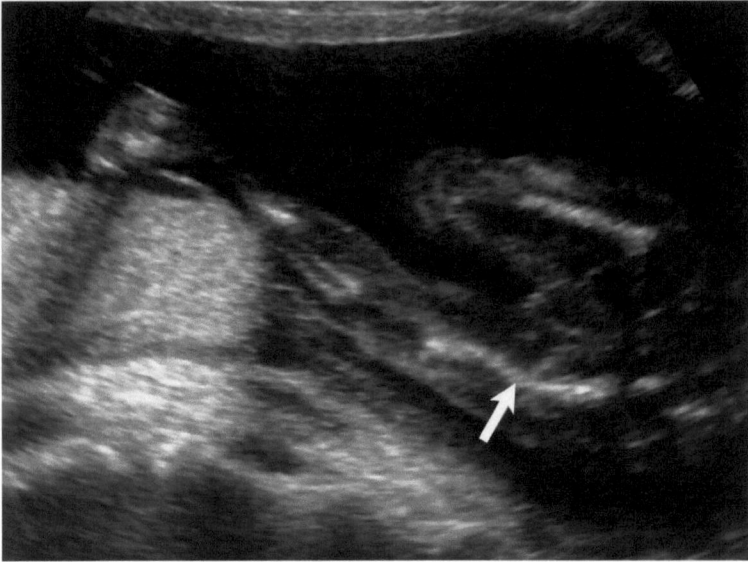

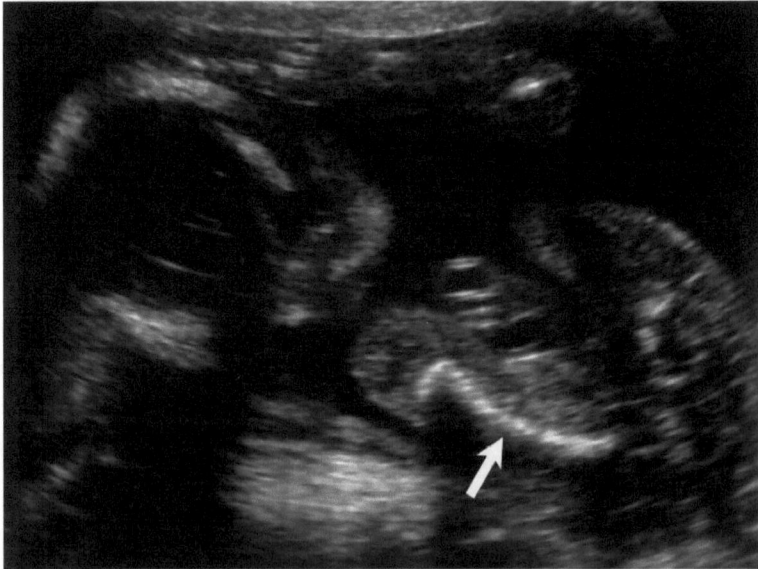

Figure 5.13: Dual image of a fetal femur shows a bowed femoral contour suggestive of a bone fracture such as can occur with osteogenesis imperfecta. The appearance is artifactual and is due to refraction. Repositioning of the transducer reveals a normal straight femur in this normal healthy mid-trimester fetus.

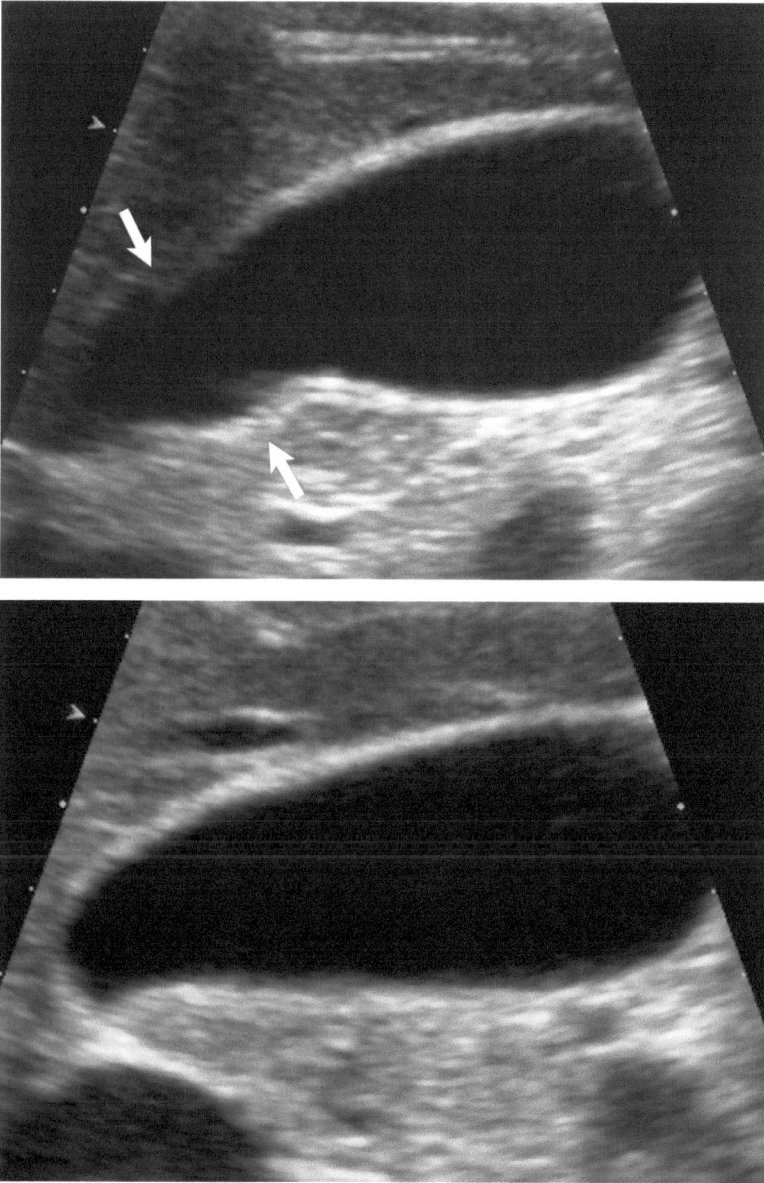

Figure 5.14: The upper image of this normal gallbladder is affected by refraction. The effect disappears after slight change of transducer position where a more uniform acoustic window exists (lower image).

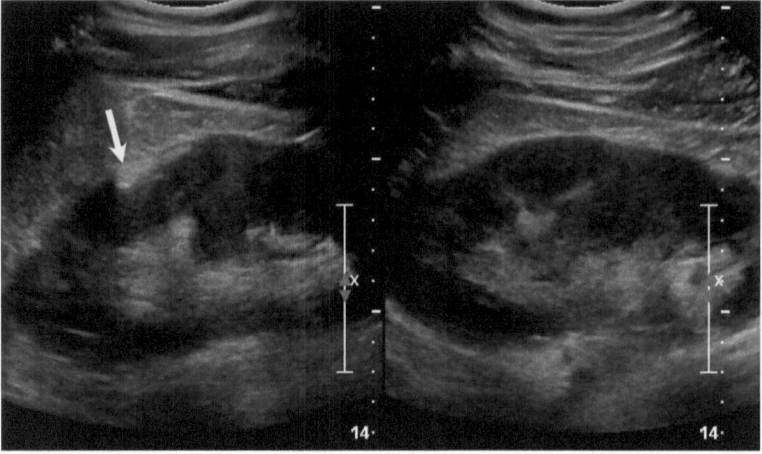

Figure 5.15: The contour abnormality seen in the upper pole of the kidney (arrow) is artifactual and is caused by a refracting rib margin. The artifact disappears after a slight change of transducer position away from the rib (right image).

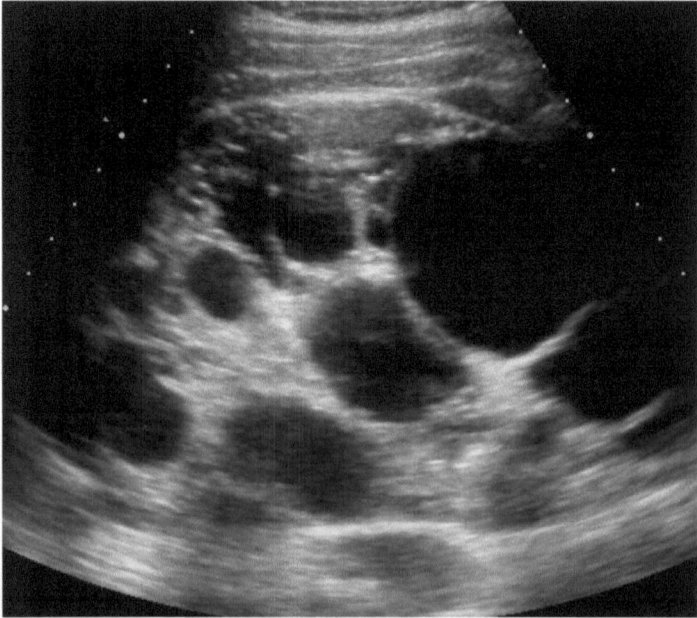

Figure 5.16: A progressive defocusing effect is seen in this patient with autosomal dominant polycystic kidney disease. Many of the cysts are fuzzy due to a range of artifacts including refraction, reverberation and beamwidth.

5.3 Anisotropy

Causative mechanisms

Anisotropy is due to variable propagation speed across and along striated structures such as muscles, tendons and ligaments. When an anisotropic structure is interrogated from an angle other than normal (90° incidence), the incident beam refracts at each interface within the structure which leads to a rapid defocusing effect manifesting as loss of echo amplitude, attenuation and dropout. The problem is well known in musculoskeletal ultrasound.

Which system assumptions have been breached?

All of the following assumptions are breached: 1) speed of sound is constant, 2) sound travels in a straight line and 3) attenuation rate is constant.

Typical appearance

Normal striated appearance of the structure of interest (muscle, tendon, ligament) at normal incidence (90°) but gradual loss of echogenicity at angles less than 90° with complete drop-out at acute angles.

Can this artifact be reduced, eliminated or circumvented?

Yes, this artifact can be eliminated if the region of interest can be scanned at normal incidence by manually angling the transducer, electronic beam-steering or the use of a favorable acoustic window. If a 90° approach is not achievable, anisotropy is difficult to eliminate. Spatial image compounding tends to reduce the effect of anisotropy because some of the beams will interrogate the region of interest at favorable angle.

Is this artifact diagnostically useful?

No. This artifact is a major problem in musculoskeletal imaging. For example, curved tendons need to be interrogated from a range of angles because some parts of the tendon will always demonstrate dropout.Less experienced practitioners can easily confuse anisotropic shadowing for real pathology such as a tendon tear.

Image examples of anisotropy are provided in the chapter on acoustic shadowing.

Chapter 6

Reverberation

Reverberation occurs when an ultrasound pulse becomes trapped between strong tissue reflectors and reflects back and forth. Each time the pulse reflects, an echo is generated. Because these echoes continue to arrive later and later, the system assumes they represent tissue reflectors from ever-increasing depth. Reverberation artifacts originating from small focal regions are known as comet-tail artifacts.

6.1 Reverberation artifact

Also known as

Not-so-amiably referred to by sonographers simply as 'reverb'.

Causative mechanisms

Two or more strong tissue reflectors are interrogated at normal incidence (90°) and the acoustic pulse becomes partially trapped by the reflectors, causing it to reflect back and forth. The causative reflectors can both be tissue reflectors or alternatively one reflector is a soft tissue reflector while the other is the transducer surface itself. Each time the pulse reflects from one of the two reflectors, an echo is generated. Because these echoes are returning to the transducer at a later and later time, the system interprets these as arriving from deeper and deeper locations and plots them progressively deeper on the display. The reverberating pulse will gradually attenuate and the artifact therefore demonstrates progressive loss of amplitude until it disappears. The reverberation artifact is most commonly caused by large horizontal reflectors encountered in the body wall including soft tissue boundaries, muscle boundaries, fascial planes, etc.

Which system assumptions have been breached?

The assumption that each reflector generates an echo only once.

Typical appearance

Horizontal bands of artifactual echoes, usually most evident in the leading (superficial) aspect of anechoic abdominal organs such as the bladder, gallbladder or other cystic masses. The reverberation artifact also often contaminates large vessels such as the carotid artery, jugular vein and others.

Can this artifact be reduced, eliminated or circumvented?

The reverberation artifact can be somewhat reduced with the reduction of gain and TGC settings, but this is not useful because real echoes in the region of reverberation (for example a soft tissue tumor on the anterior bladder wall) will be reduced as well. The most effective ways of reducing reverberation are:

1   Tilting the transducer in the scan plane or elevation plane so that it is not incident to the reverberating structures at 90°.

2   Relaxing the transducer pressure. With the application of transducer pressure, tissue planes are more likely to line up and form reverberating interfaces. Reverberation also tends to weaken and vanish with distance. Relaxing the transducer pressure may expand the soft tissue and increase the distance from the causative structures to the structure of interest enough for reverberation to diminish.

3   Using tissue harmonic imaging (THI). Because harmonic frequencies need time/distance to develop, few harmonics are produced in the body wall and few reverberating harmonics are

therefore produced. It is sometimes said that harmonics 'bypass' the abdominal wall.

4   Spatial compound imaging may help to average out the artifact since at least some of the ultrasound beams are not at 90° to the reverberating interfaces.

5   Using another acoustic window which contains more homogeneous tissues (if available). For example in gynecologic imaging, switching from a transabdominal to a transvaginal approach allows the operator to bypass the abdominal wall altogether.

6   If the artifactual echoes are difficult to separate from real echoes, inducing movement of the target structure by manual compression or asking the patient to breathe in will reveal movement of the target structure whereas the location of reverberation remains fixed.

Is this artifact diagnostically useful?

No. Reverberation is never useful.

Examples

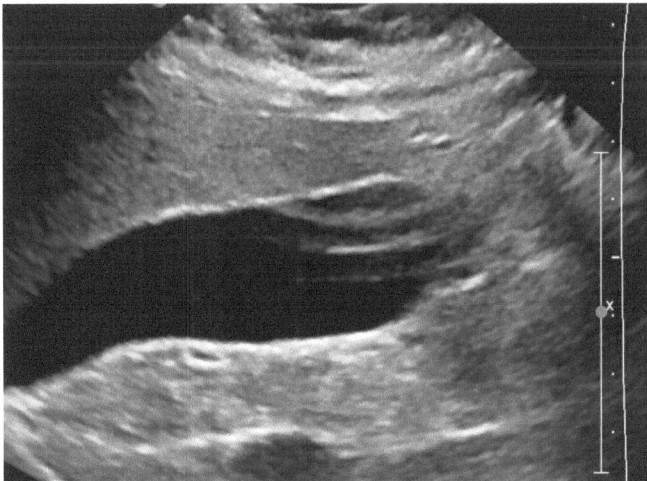

Figure 6.1: Example showing prominent reverberation artifact in the fundus of the gallbladder.

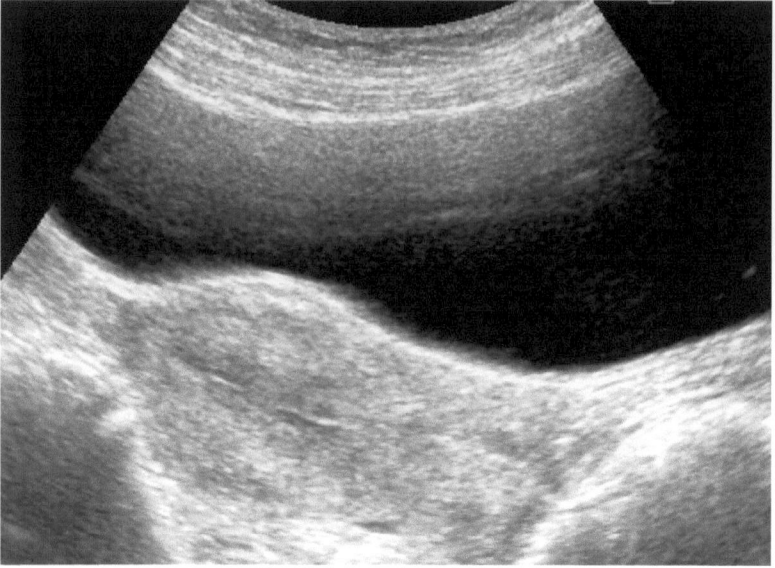

Figure 6.2: Prominent reverberation artifact in the urinary bladder.

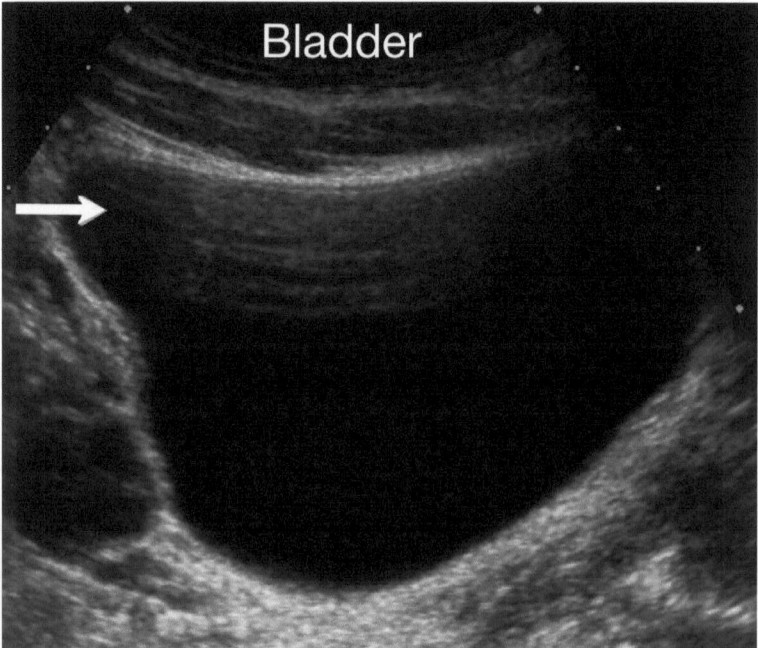

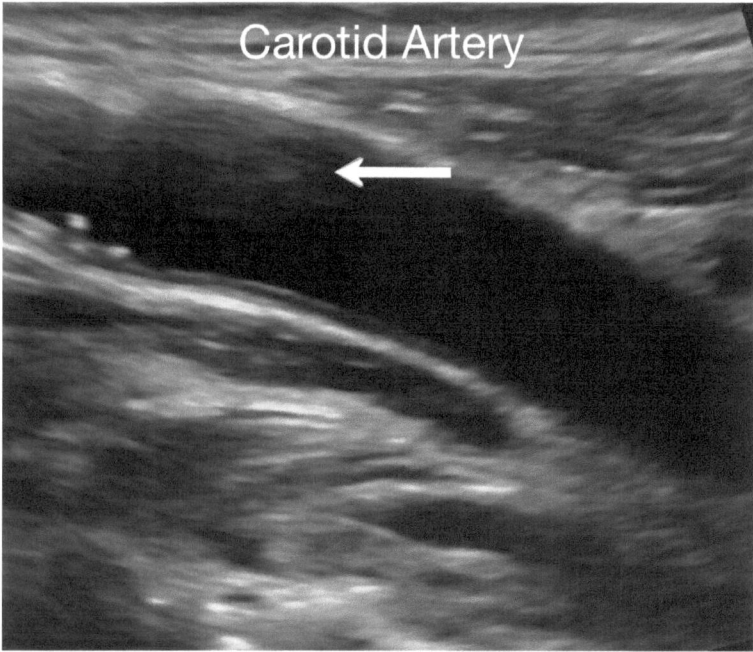

Carotid Artery

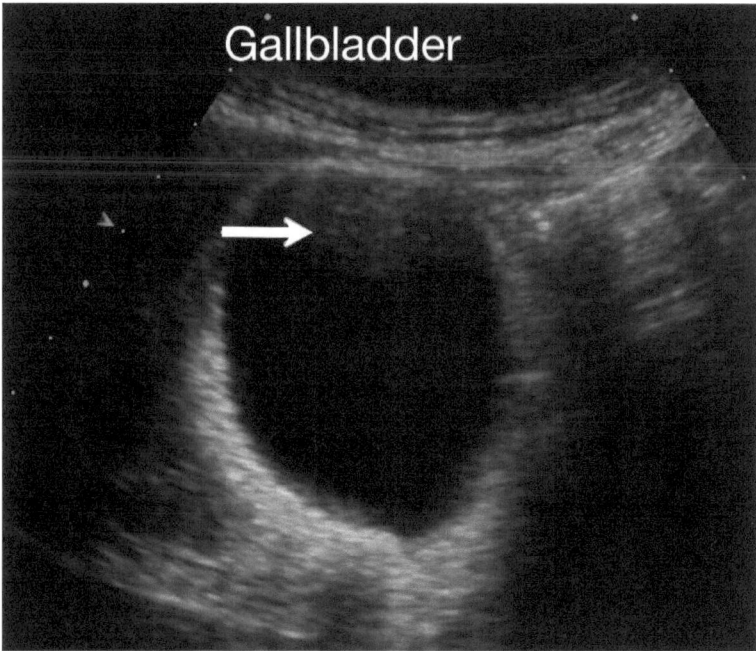

Gallbladder

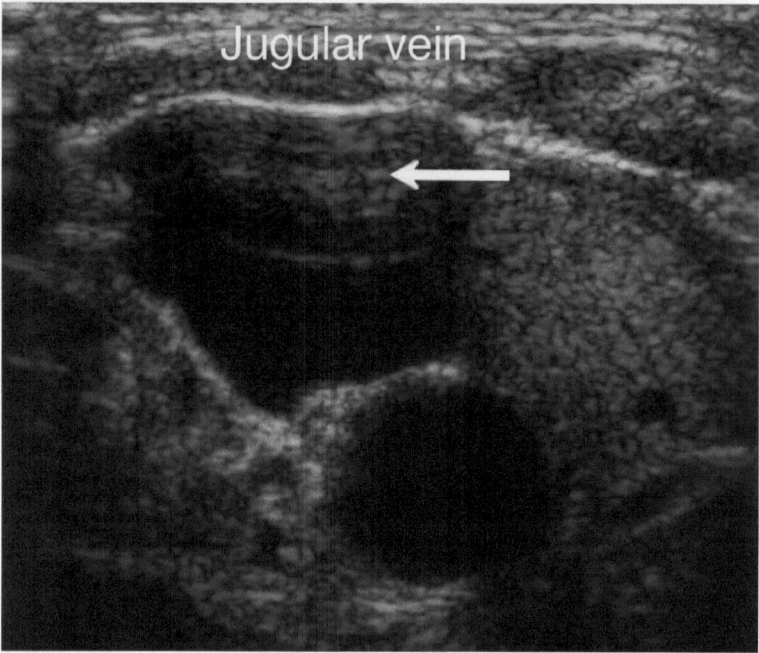

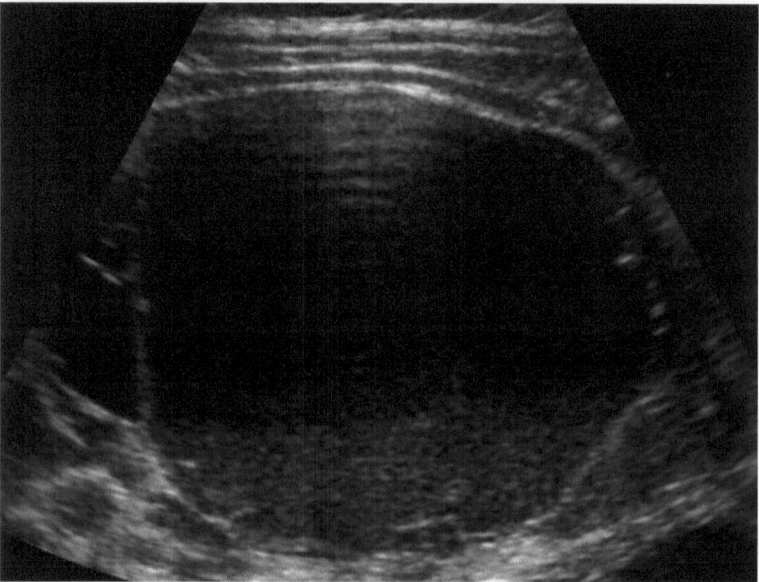

Figure 6.3: *Reverberation within a large renal cyst containing some low level particulate debris.*

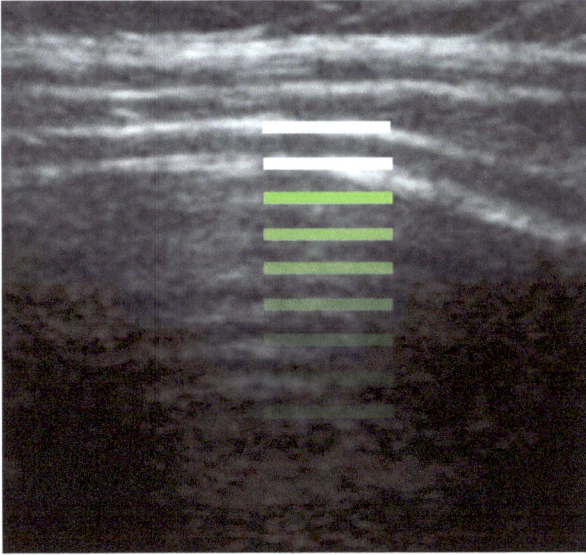

Figure 6.4: An enlarged version of the image in Figure 6.3. The causative interfaces are highlighted in white. Note that the reverberation artifact has identical spacing. As the amplitude of the reverberating pulse diminishes over time, the artifact also disappears with time/depth (green lines).

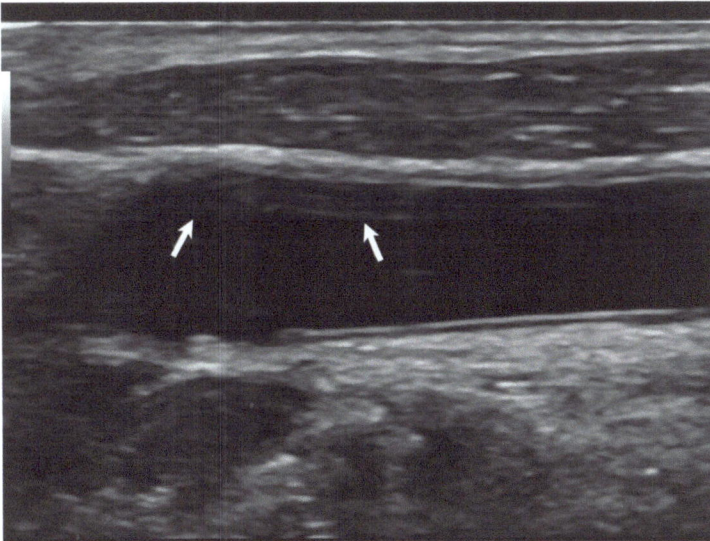

Figure 6.5: In this image, reverberation artifact is mimicking carotid plaque or thrombus.

Reverberation artifact: effect of transducer pressure

The reverberation artifact tends to weaken with time/depth. Increasing the distance between the causative structure and the structure of interest may substantially reduce the effect of reverberation.

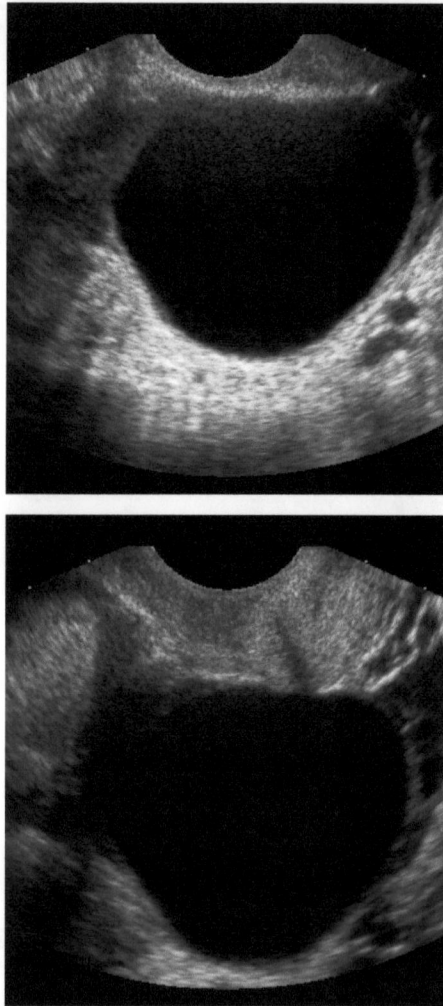

Figure 6.6: Reverberation artifact is seen contaminating the leading portion of this simple ovarian cyst (upper image). The artifact is not apparent and contrast resolution improves after the sonographer reduced transducer pressure (lower image).

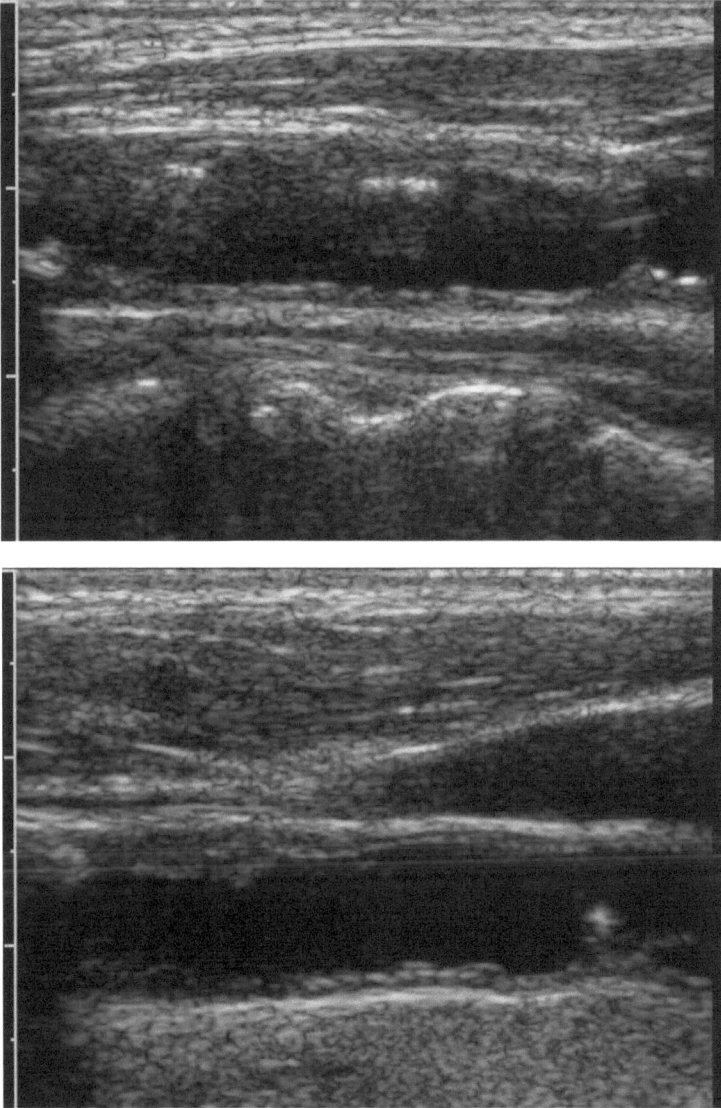

Figure 6.7: The reverberation artifact often affects visualization of vessels. In this example, reverberation artifact is seen contaminating the lumen of the common carotid artery (CCA) in the top image. The artifact is not apparent and contrast resolution improves after the sonographer reduces transducer pressure (lower image). In this case, the added advantage of reducing pressure is that the structure of interest (CCA) lies closer to the elevation plane focus of this transducer where slice thickness is smaller.

Reverberation artifact: angle dependence

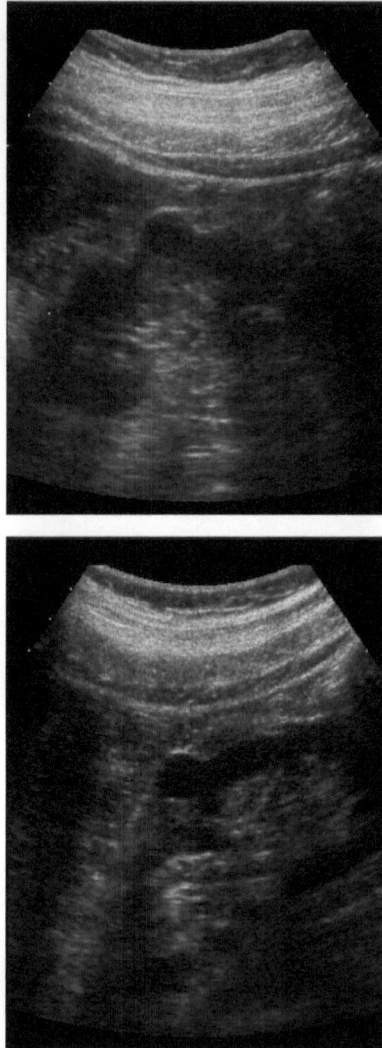

Figure 6.8: The reverberation artifact is seen filling the lumen of a simple cyst when the transducer is perpendicular to the abdominal wall (upper image) giving the impression of a solid mass. Reduction of reverberation and improvement in contrast resolution was achieved by tilting (heel-toeing) the transducer in the scan plane away from 90° (lower image). Tilting the transducer away from 90° incidence to the abdominal wall in the scan plane or elevation plane or both tends to reduce reverberation.

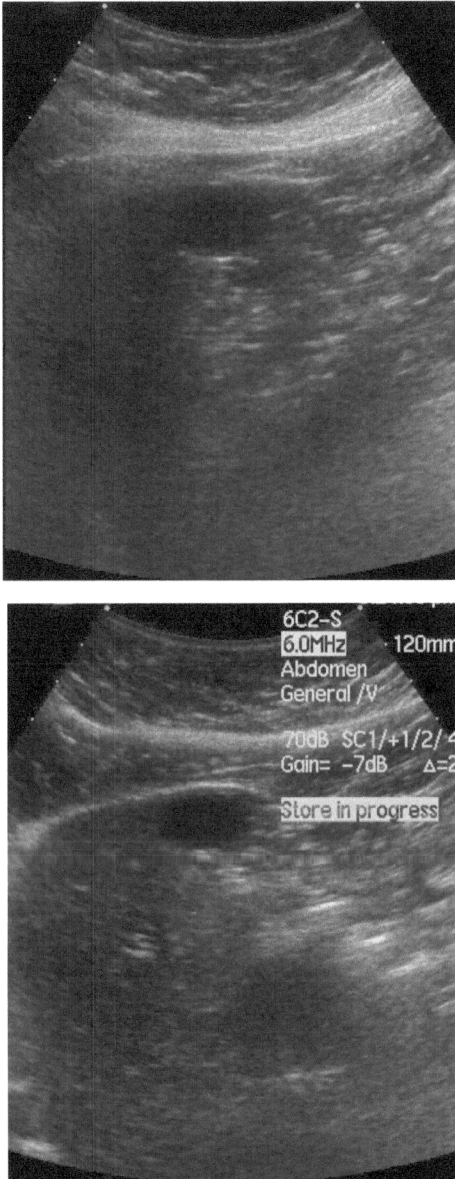

Figure 6.9: The reverberation artifact is seen filling the lumen of a simple cyst when the transducer is directed perpendicular to the abdominal wall (upper image). In this case, reduction of reverberation and improvement in contrast resolution was achieved by tilting the transducer away from 90° in the elevation plane (lower image).

Reverberation artifacts and solid structures

Reverberation artifacts tend to produce echoes of low amplitude. The artifact is easy to spot in anechoic structures but it blends into solid organs such as the liver where it degrades image quality while being rather inconspicuous. The artifact may reduce the operator's ability to visualize real objects in the zone of reverberation, however, the operator may be unaware the artifact is there. Can you determine which image in this liver series is most affected by reverberation?

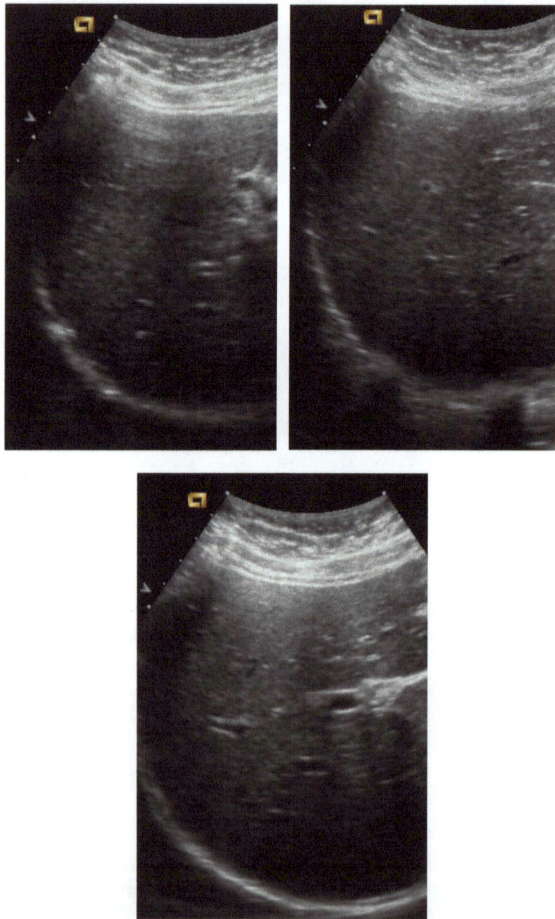

Figure 6.10: The upper left image is particularly degraded by reverberation. A small mass in the superficial portion of the liver would not be detectable.

6.2 Comet tail artifact

Causative mechanisms

Similar to reverberation, two or more strong tissue reflectors are interrogated at normal incidence (90°) and the acoustic pulse becomes partially trapped by the reflectors causing it to reflect back and forth. What separates comet tail artifact from large scale reverberation is the small focal nature of the reflectors and therefore narrow width of the artifact. The comet tail artifact is often seen in adenomyomatosis/cholesterolosis of the gallbladder where cholesterol crystals in the mucosal folds of the gallbladder form reflective interfaces that promote the artifact's formation.

Which system assumptions have been breached?

The assumption that each reflector generates an echo only once.

Typical appearance

Small stalactite-like artifacts projecting along lines of sight into otherwise anechoic regions.

Can this artifact be reduced, eliminated or circumvented?

Comet tail artifacts are usually persistent and are difficult to eliminate. Fortunately due to their small size, they rarely pose a major problem for adequate assessment of the target structure. The usual methods of reducing reverberation often fail to reduce this artifact completely. Spatial compounding tends to reduce the length of the comet tail. With large comet tail artifacts, a different angle of approach can help change the artifact's position and allow visualization of structures previously obscured by the artifact.

Is this artifact diagnostically useful?

Since this artifact is characteristically associated with certain pathologies such as adenomyomatosis/cholesterolosis and colloid thyroid nodules, it is diagnostically useful in these specific circumstances.

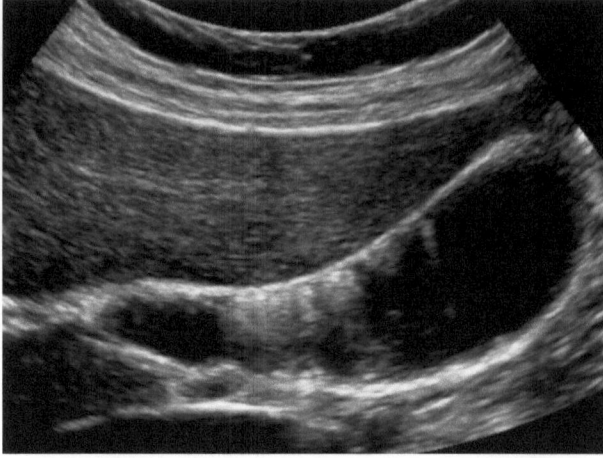

Figure 6.11: Classic appearance of adenomyomatosis of the gallbladder wall with numerous comet tail artifacts.

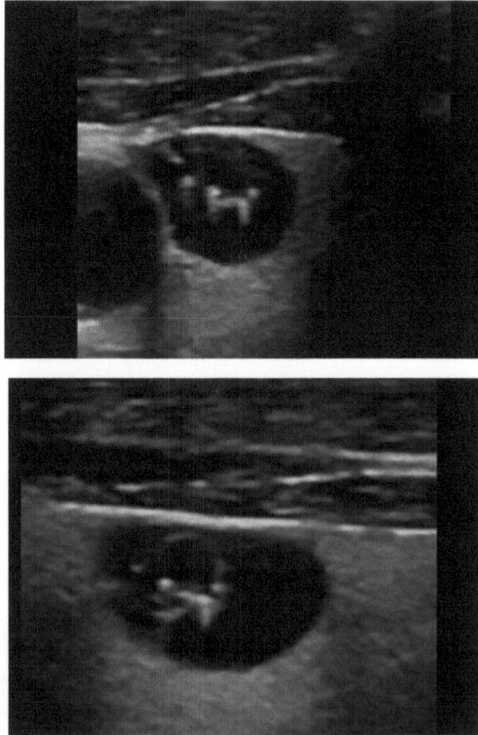

Figure 6.12: Colloid cysts in the thyroid often demonstrate comet tail artifacts.

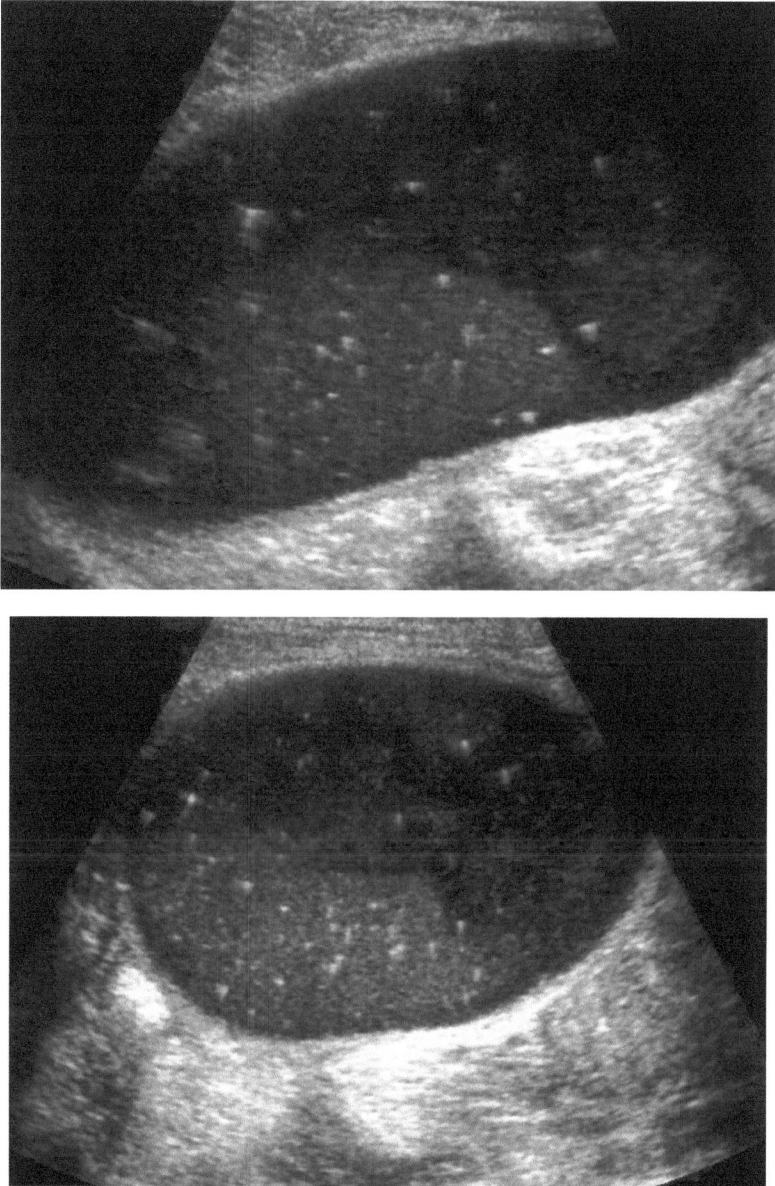

Figure 6.13: Sludge-filled gallbladder with floating cholesterol crystals which occasionally line up in a favorable configuration to cause comet tail artifacts.

Comet tail artifacts can be associated with sutures, prosthetic material and foreign bodies.

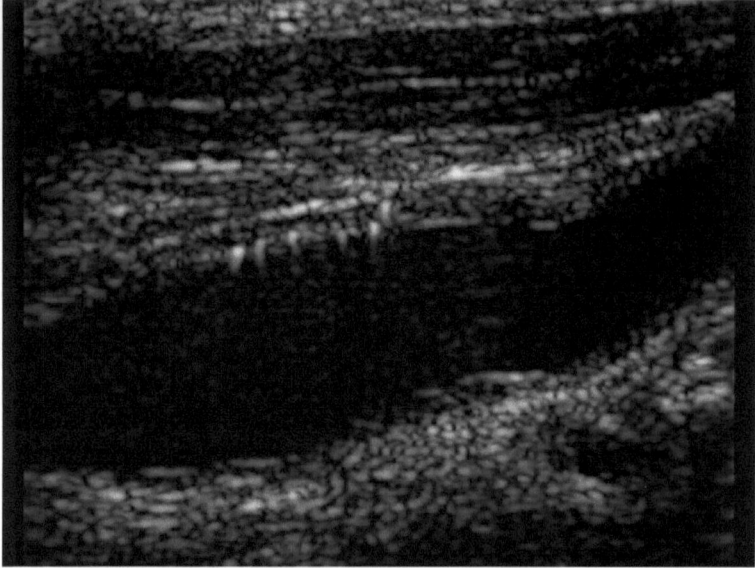

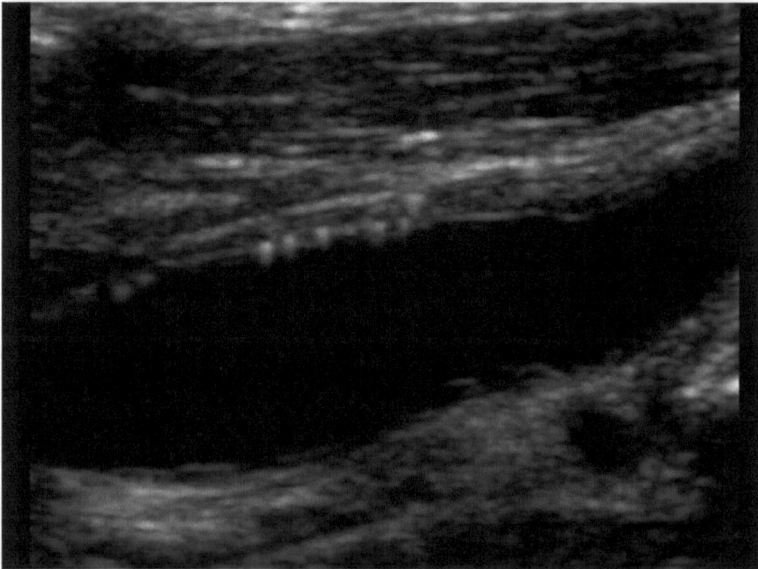

Figure 6.14: In this image, numerous small comet tail artifacts are associated with a carotid endarterectomy patch. Note the artifact is slightly larger in the non-compounded image (top) than the compounded image (bottom).

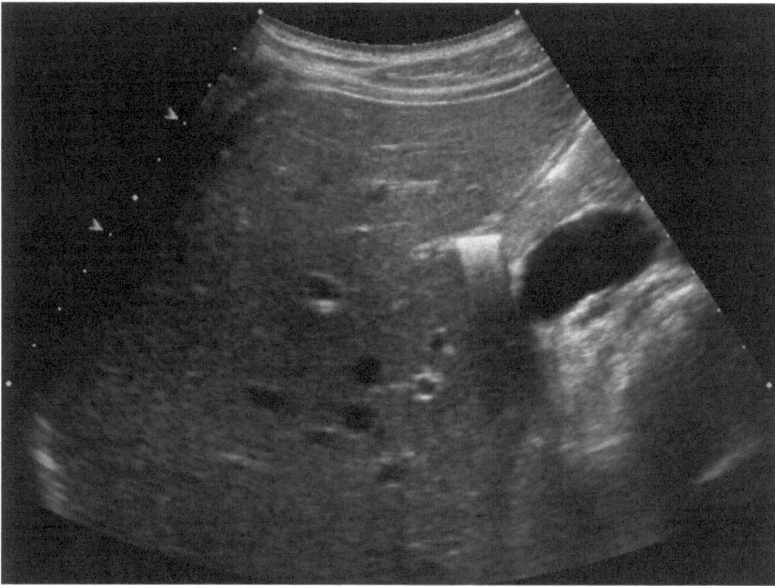

Figure 6.15: Wider comet tail artifact and dirty shadowing are associated with a surgical clip in this patient post cholecystectomy.

Chapter 7

Ringdown

The ringdown artifact is classically associated with gas. It can also be seen with metal such as foreign bodies and needles. Ringdown is a prominent artifact which appears as streams of high amplitude echoes all the way to the bottom of the image.

Causative mechanisms

For ringdown to occur, high amplitude echoes need to be produced continuously after the incident ultrasound pulse strikes the causative structure. This can occur when the ultrasound beam encounters a cluster of gas bubbles. Gas bubbles act as elastic bodies and they can vibrate or resonate in the ultrasound beam. Ringdown is also sometimes seen in association with metal (foreign bodies, needles, surgical staples) because these structures continue to 'ring' after the acoustic pulse has gone through.

Which system assumptions have been breached?

The assumption that each reflector produces an echo only once.

Typical appearance

Individual streaks or entire curtains of high amplitude echoes emanating from the causative structure along the line of sight.

If associated with bowel gas, peristalsis will change the location of the artifact in the image.

Common misconceptions

Students of ultrasound often confuse reverberation and ringdown. The two are quite distinct artifacts in their causation and appearance. Ringdown is characterized by its high amplitude and lack of attenuation with distance. In contrast, reverberation demonstrates diminishing echo amplitude.

Can this artifact be reduced, eliminated or circumvented?

If the causative agent is gas, then graded compression may help displace the bowel gas and allow visualization of deeper structures. Other forms of ringdown cannot be eliminated.

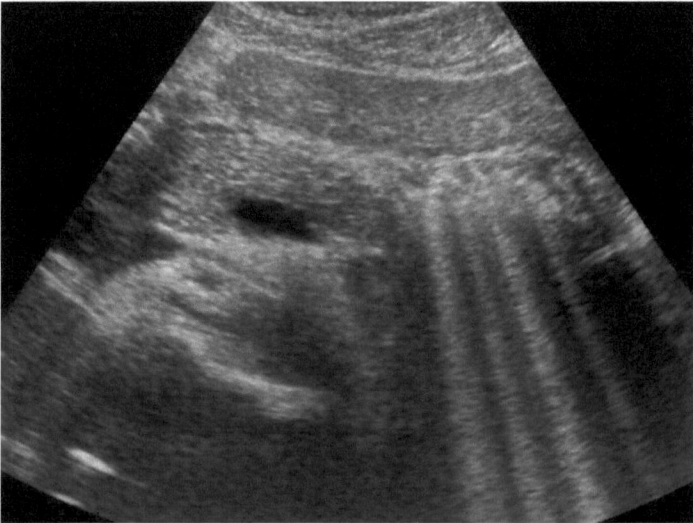

Figure 7.1: Prominent ringdown artifact associated with normal bowel gas.

Is this artifact diagnostically useful?

Ringdown can be useful in some clinical scenarios. For example, it tends to suggest the presence of gas within organs which can be useful as a diagnostic clue in conditions ranging from pneumobilia, gangrenous cholecystitis and other infected regions and abscesses containing air.

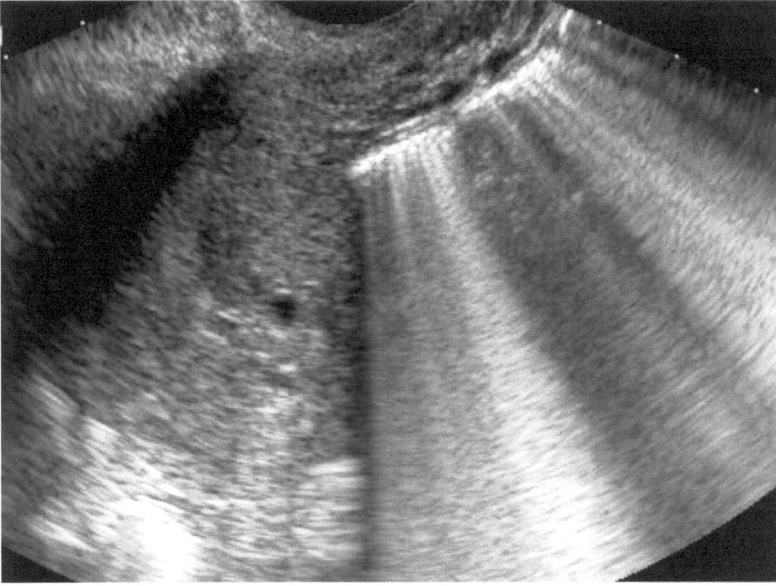

Figure 7.2: A second example of ringdown artifact associated with normal bowel gas.

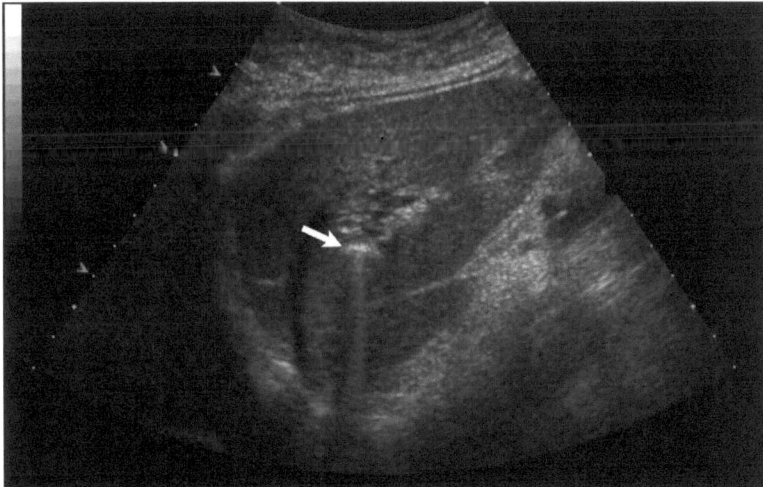

Figure 7.3: The presence of ring-down behind the small echogenic intrahepatic focus in this patient with mild biliary dilation post ERCP confirms the presence of pneumobilia. Otherwise, the differential diagnosis would also need to include a Von Meyenburg complex, an intraductal calculus, a granuloma or a calcification.

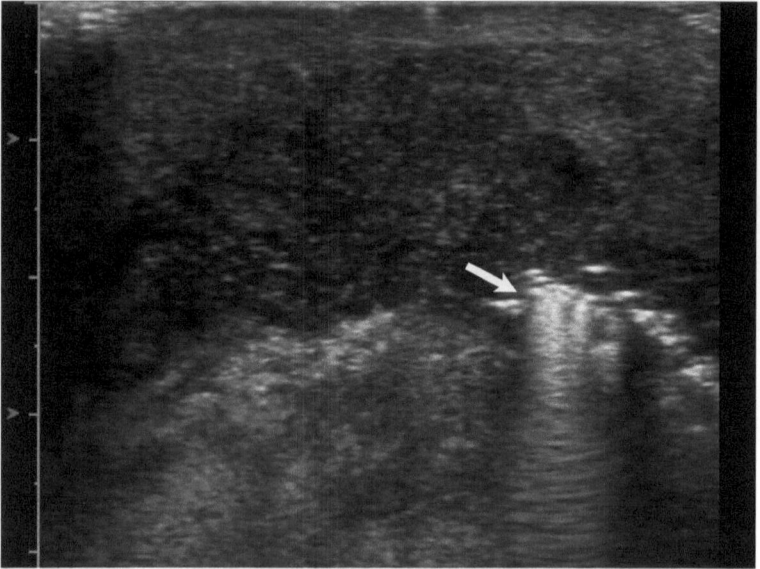

Figure 7.4: Scrotal wall abscess in a diabetic patient demonstrates the presence of gas bubbles with ringdown artifacts.

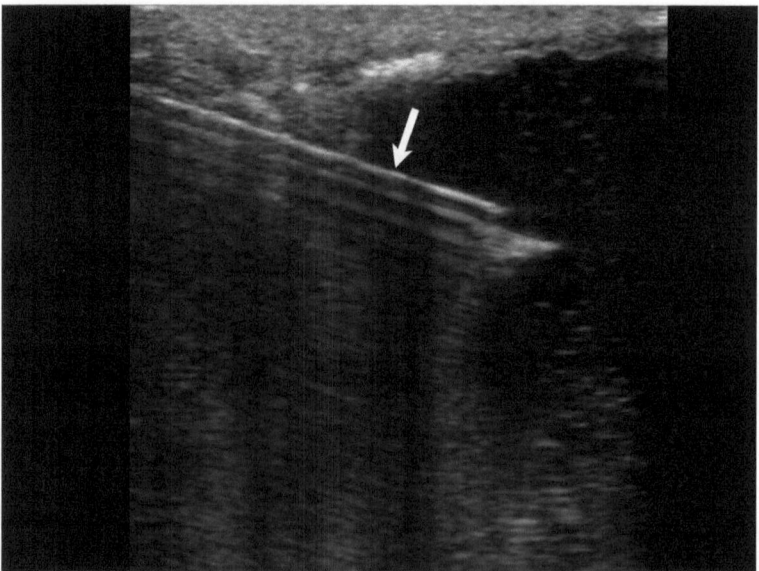

Figure 7.5: A ringdown artifact associated with a needle used for percutaneous drainage of a fluid collection.

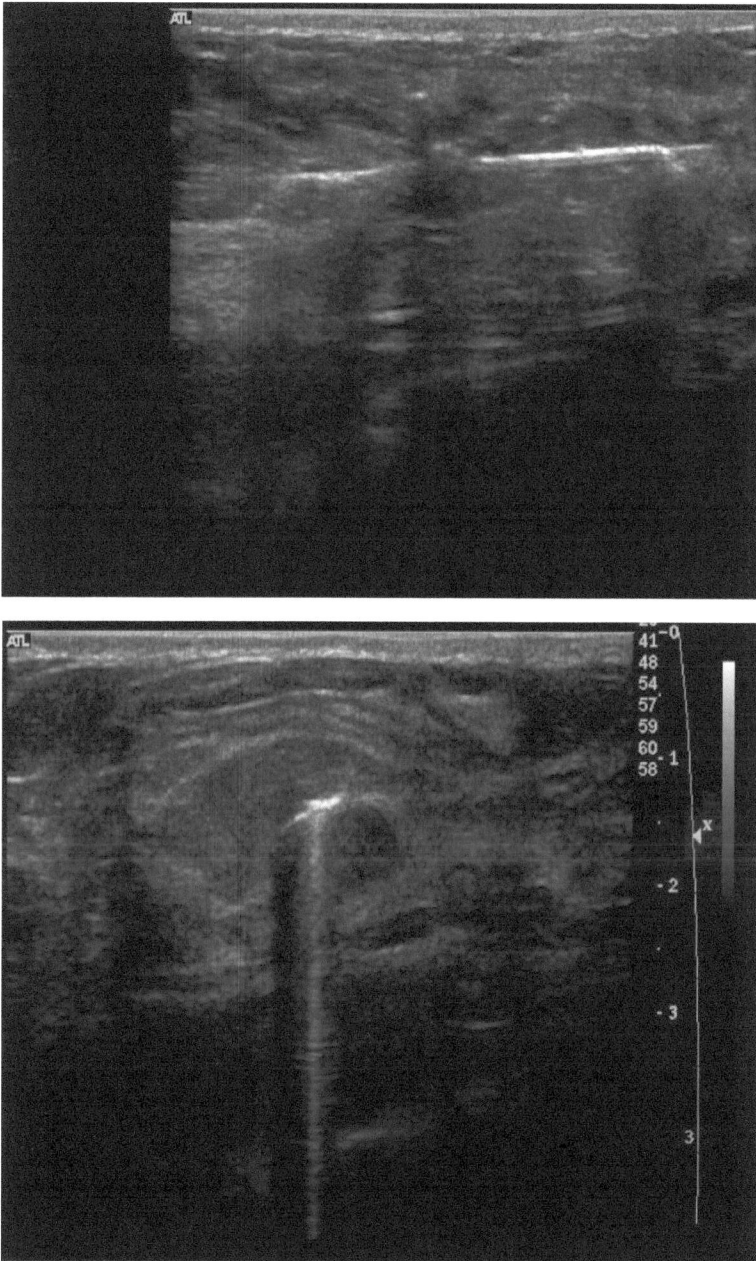

Figure 7.6: The ringdown artifact is seen in a transverse view of a breast biopsy needle (lower image). It is not apparent in the longitudinal section (upper image) in this case.

Chapter 8

Mirror Image Artifacts

> Mirror image artifacts occur when the ultrasound beam encounters large specular reflectors which act as acoustic mirrors rather than scatterers. A wide range of interesting and potentially confusing appearances can be seen in association with acoustic mirrors.

Causative mechanisms

Mirror image artifacts occur when the ultrasound beam encounters a large specular reflector which acts as an acoustic mirror. Mirrors tend to reflect ultrasound pulses so that the angle of incidence equals the angle of reflection. There are many types of acoustic mirrors including:

1   Pleura/air interface seen beyond the diaphragm in transabdominal views of the liver and spleen. Pleura/air mirror can also be seen in views of subclavian structures when the apex of the lung is in the field of view.

2   Bowel wall/bowel gas interface. This mirror is especially known to affect the region of the rectum in transabdominal views of the bladder and recto-vessical region particularly in children.

3   Flat bone surfaces such as parts of the tibia, skull (fetal and adult).

4   Flat layers of calcium such as calcified arterial wall seen in cases

of diabetic arteriopathy (medial calcification) or diffuse calcific atheromatous plaques.

5   Deep (investing) fascia of muscles sometimes acts as acoustic mirror.

Which system assumptions have been breached?

The assumption that the beam path is straight.

Typical appearance

Acoustic mirrors are always highly reflective and therefore intensely echogenic interfaces. For a mirror image artifact to be present, the mirror must be present within the field of view. If an operator believes the image is being affected by a mirror image artifact, it is important that the operator identifies the mirror. Classic textbook descriptions of mirror image artifacts usually involve apparent duplication of objects with the true object in front of the acoustic mirror and the false object behind the mirror. In clinical ultrasound, however, mirror image phenomena are rarely this straightforward. Depending on the tilt, curvature, surface irregularity and acoustic opacity of the mirror (complete versus partial mirror), the false object may be a different size, shape, echotexture and may appear in a different plane of section to the original object. In general, if the mirror is relatively straight and flat, the false object will be of similar size and shape to the original object. If the mirror is concave, the false object will appear larger. If the mirror is convex, the false object will appear smaller.

Common misconceptions

There are a number of commonly held misconceptions regarding mirror image artifacts:

- *Misconception 1: the false object will be identical in size, shape and echotexture to the true object.* This is not the case.

- *Misconception 2: the false object is always visible alongside the original object.* This is not true because a tilted mirror may project the false object into a different plane. Imagine looking into a bathroom mirror. You will only see your reflection if you are looking into the mirror at normal incidence. If the mirror is tilted away from normal in any plane, your image will be projected elsewhere.

- *Misconception 3: if a structure of similar echotexture to a true object exists where mirror image artifacts often occur, that structure can safely be assumed to represent a false object from a mirror image artifact.* This assumption is a diagnostic trap and is clinically dangerous. For instance, some lung pathologies for example large solid tumors, empyema, hemothorax and others may produce echotexture highly reminiscent of liver characteristics.

- *Misconception 4: the diaphragm causes mirror image artifacts to occur.* The diaphragm is a muscular organ and is no different in its acoustic properties to other muscles around the body. Clinical experience will reveal the fact that muscles do not act as acoustic mirrors, yet the diaphragm is often blamed for causing mirror image artifacts. The true mirror is not the diaphragm but rather the pleura/air interface beyond the diaphragm. It is air in the lung that creates an acoustic mirror. This is why mirror image artifacts are not observed in patients with pleural effusions.

Can this artifact be reduced, eliminated or circumvented?

In general it is not possible to eliminate this artifact, but it may be possible to circumvent it by using a different angle of approach or different acoustic window.

Is this artifact diagnostically useful?

Apart from being academically interesting, mirror image artifacts are never clinically useful and can lead to confusing images. There are several helpful strategies that can assist the operator to distinguish a mirror image from true pathology:

1 Is there are mirror in the image? Mirrors are always highly echogenic.

2 Can normal structures be seen in the dependent part of the image? If yes, the image is not a mirror image artifact because it is generally not possible to see through a mirror.

3 Can the structure be seen from another acoustic window?

Mirror image artifact: examples

Mirror: pleura/air interface

The best known mirror image artifact involves the apparent projection of the liver into the region of the chest.

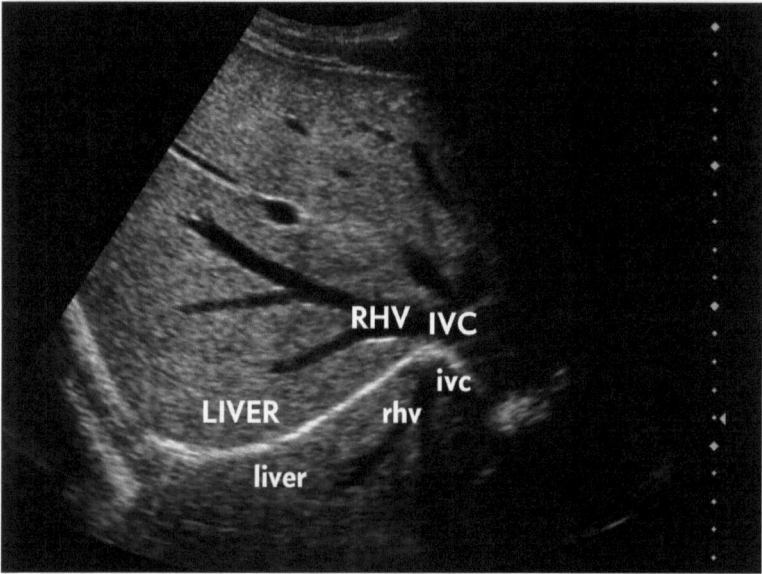

Figure 8.1: In this image the liver parenchyma, right hepatic vein (RHV) and Inferior Vena Cava (IVC) are all mirrored. The true objects are labelled in capital letters with the corresponding mirrored objects in lower case.

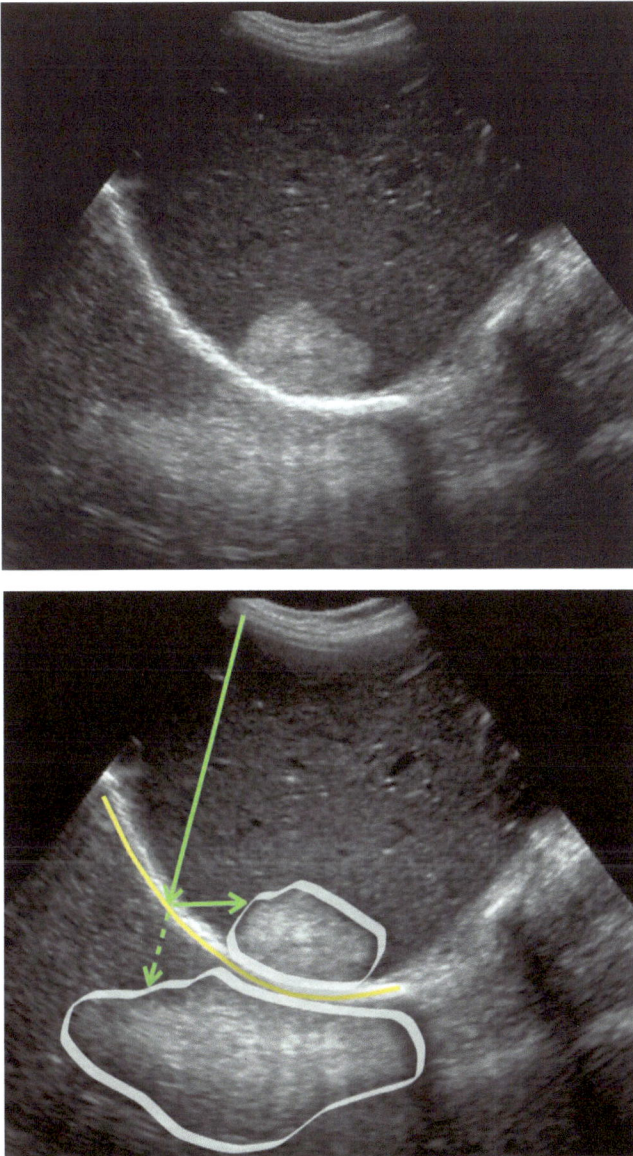

Figure 8.2: Mirror image of a liver hemangioma is seen projected into the chest (upper image). Note that the false object appears much larger than the original object due to the effect of mirror curvature. The true and assumed beam paths which lead to the apparent "stretching" of the hemangioma are shown in the lower diagram (true beam path solid arrows; assumed beam path dithered arrow, acoustic mirror yellow highlight).

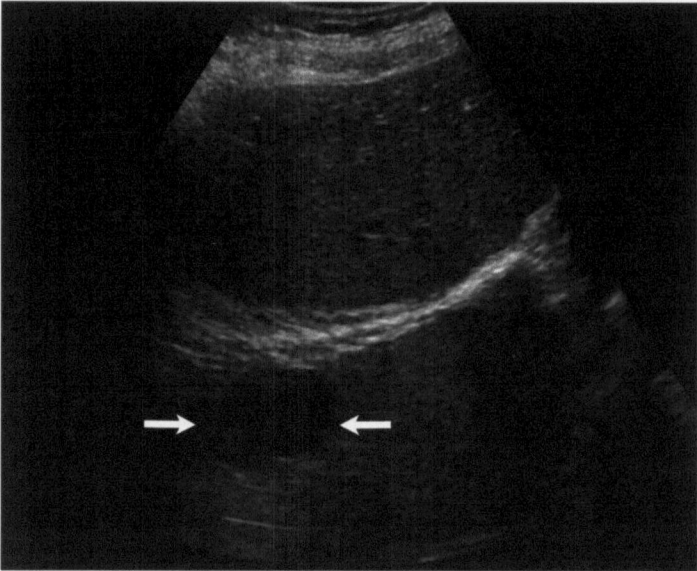

Figure 8.3: A mirror which is tilted out of plane may result in the visualization of a mirrored object without the visualization of the true object. In this example, a liver cyst is being projected into the chest. The true object is not visualized. It lies within the liver either in front or behind the current plane of section.

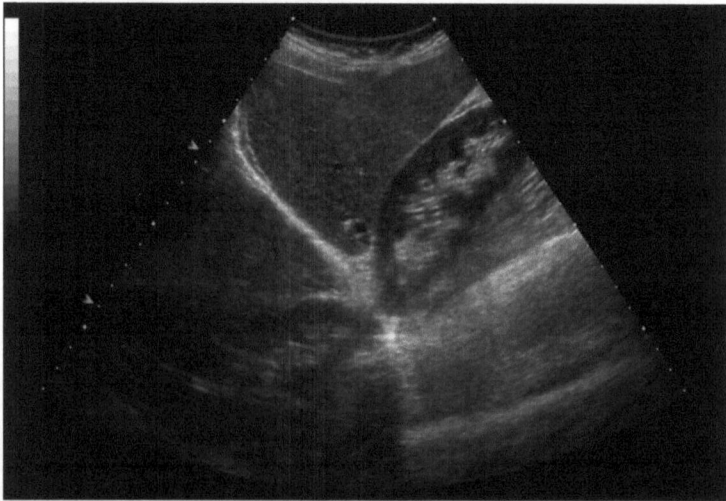

Figure 8.4: The liver and kidney are being mirrored in this image of the right upper quadrant (RUQ). Both the true objects and the false (mirror) objects are visualized.

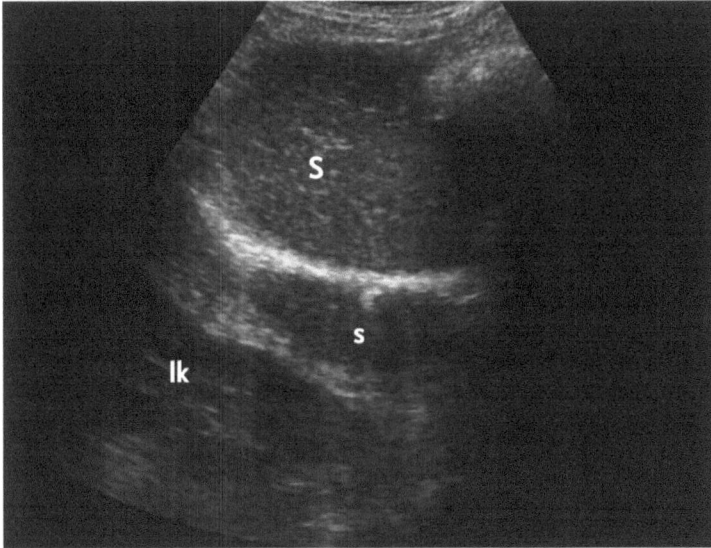

Figure 8.5: The left kidney and parts of the spleen are being mirrored in this image. However, due to the tilt of the acoustic mirror, one of the true objects (left kidney) is not visualized. The spleen (S) and the mirror image of the spleen (s) are both seen, but are different in shape.

Mirror: fetal skulls

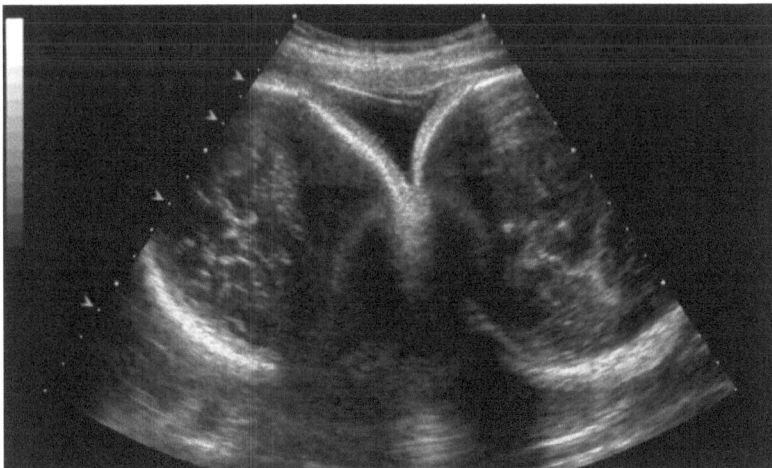

Figure 8.6: Live twin gestation showing reciprocal projections of the skull margin into each twin's skull.

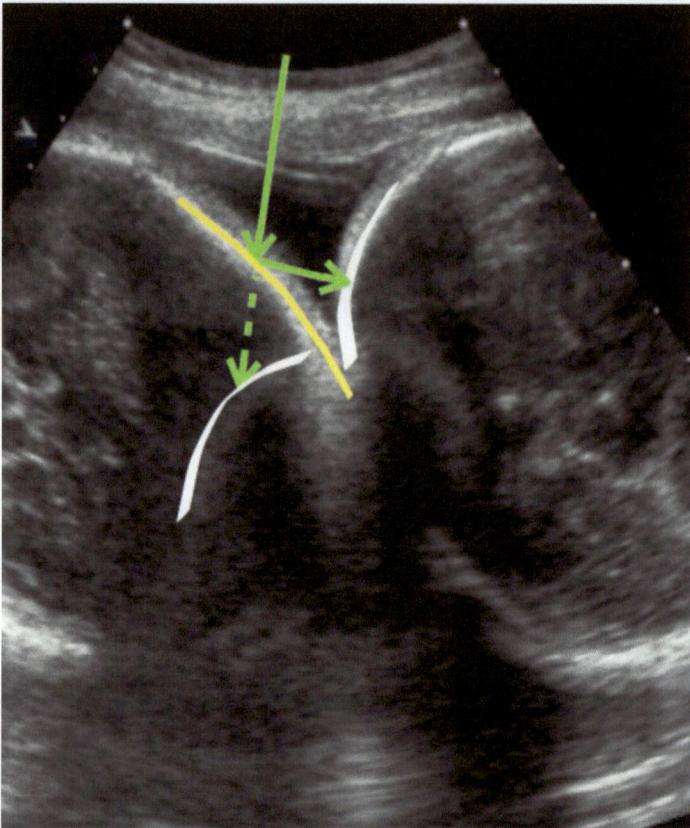

Figure 8.7: The true and assumed beam paths which lead to one of the artifacts shown in Figure 8.6 (true beam path solid arrows, assumed beam path dithered arrows, acoustic mirror yellow highlight).

Mirror 1: tibial surface, Mirror 2: transducer surface

This type of mirroring, where multiple copies of the same object are seen, can occur when two opposing mirrors reflect the same object back and forth. Some hotel elevators have mirrors on opposing walls leading to an interesting optical illusion of multiple copies of the occupants disappearing into infinity.

In the case of the image shown in Figures 8.8 and 8.9, the tibial surface forms one mirror and the opposing mirror is the transducer surface. One can think of this image as an exceptionally good form of reverberation where the specular reflectors as well as the soft tissue are being replicated.

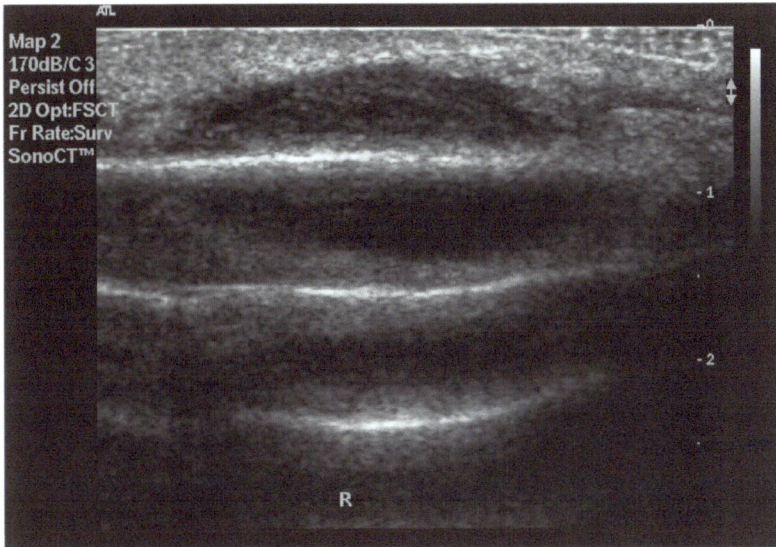

Figure 8.8: A pre-tibial hematoma is being assessed using a linear array transducer. There are several copies of the mass below the tibial surface.

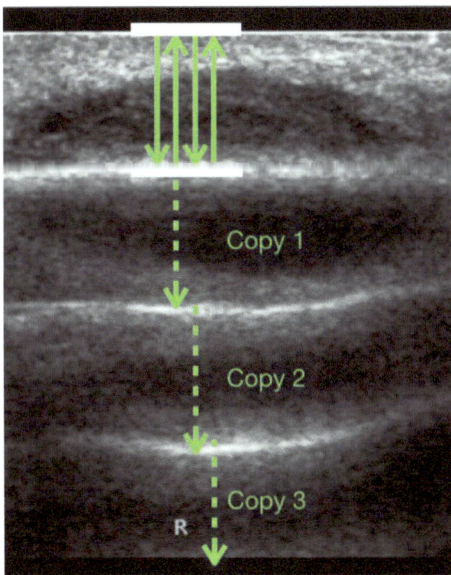

Figure 8.9: The true and assumed beam paths for the image shown in Figure 8.8 (true beam path solid arrows, assumed beam path dithered arrows).

Mirror: tibial surface

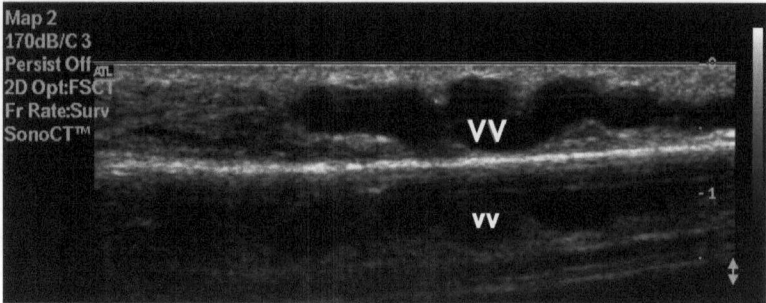

Figure 8.10: Pre-tibial varicose vein (VV) with corresponding mirror image artifact below the tibial surface (vv).

Mirror: lung air

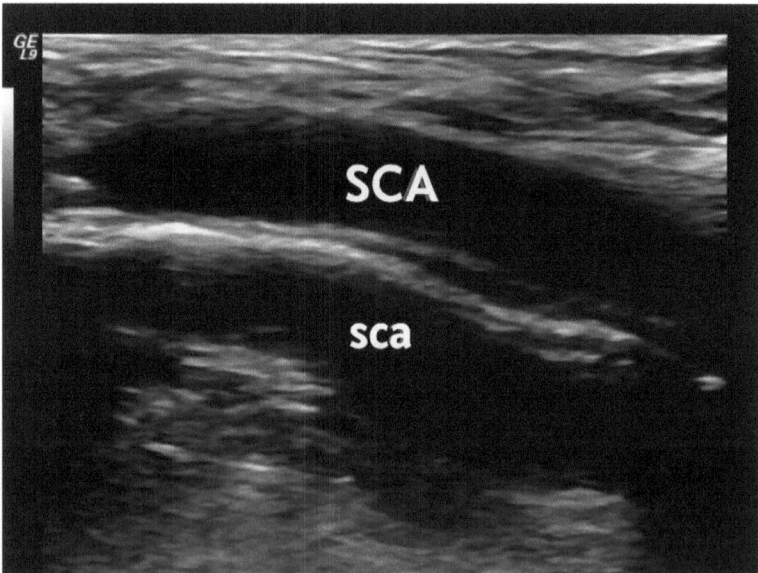

Figure 8.11: The subclavian artery (SCA) and its mirror image (sca) are visualized in the infraclavicular window.

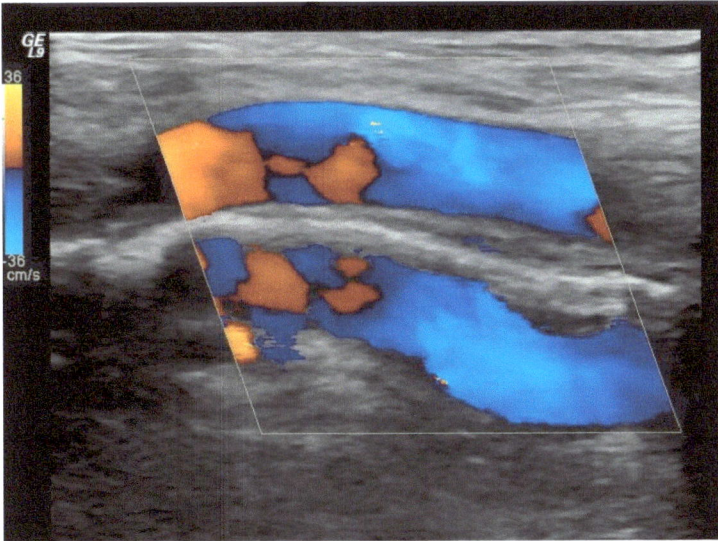

Figure 8.12: The mirror effect can be visualized in all imaging modes including color Doppler (see above), and also power Doppler and spectral Doppler.

Mirror: tracheal air

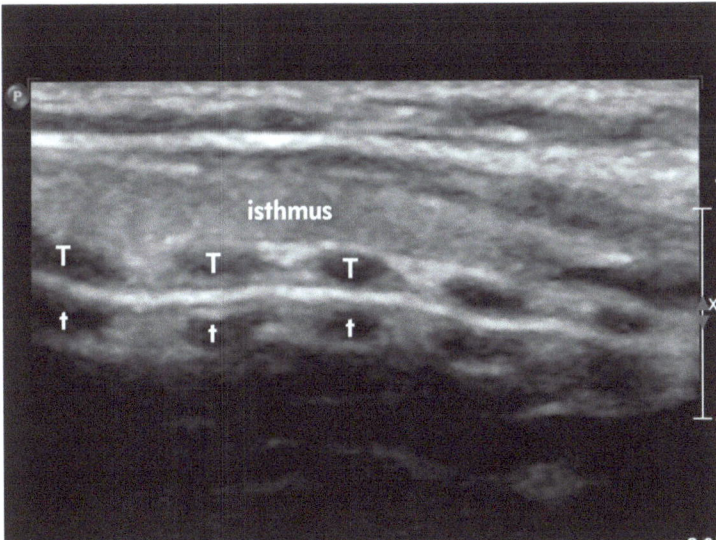

Figure 8.13: Mid-sagittal image of the thyroid isthmus demonstrates the cartilaginous rings of the trachea (T) with corresponding mirror images (t).

Mirror: rectal gas

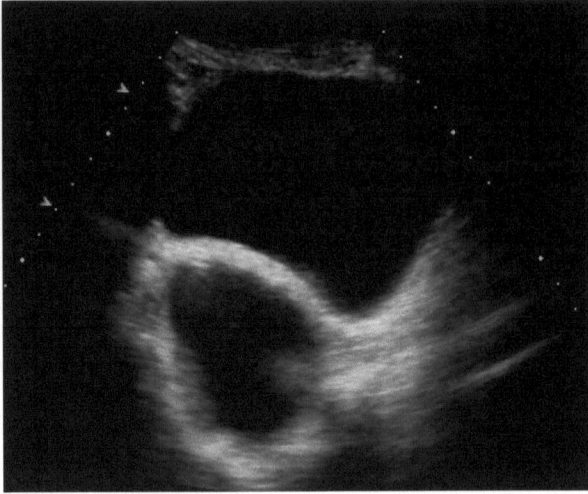

Figure 8.14: This mirror image artifact of the bladder mimics a cystic pelvic mass. The mirror has a convex curvature with respect to the incident beam causing the false object to appear smaller than the original object.

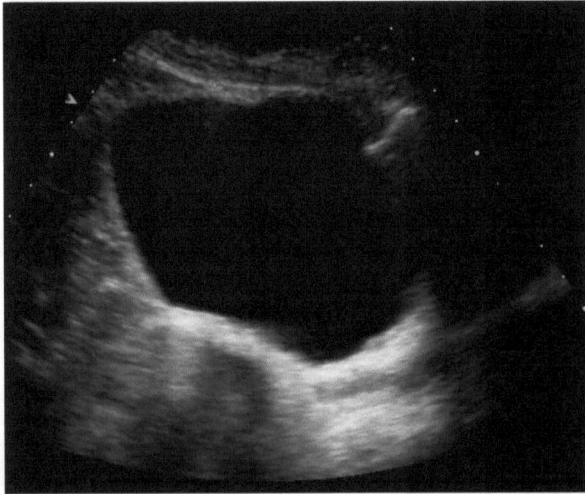

Figure 8.15: The same patient as shown in Figure 8.14. A small change in the angle of approach caused the mirror image artifact to disappear.

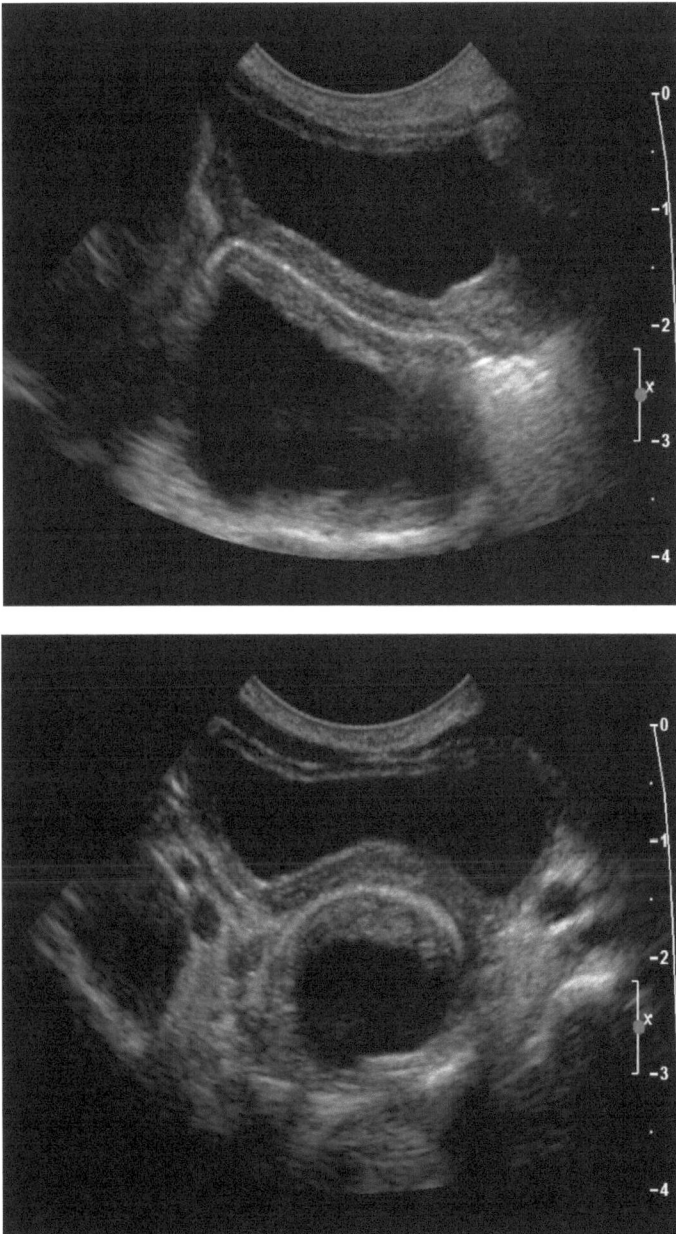

Images courtesy Roger Gent, Adelaide. Reproduced by permission.

Figure 8.16: Another example of a mirror image artifact mimicking a pelvic mass. The artifact is present both in longitudinal and transverse views.

Separating fact from mirror image artifact

Are the echoes above the diaphragm in this patient real or artifactual (see Figures 8.17 and 8.18)?

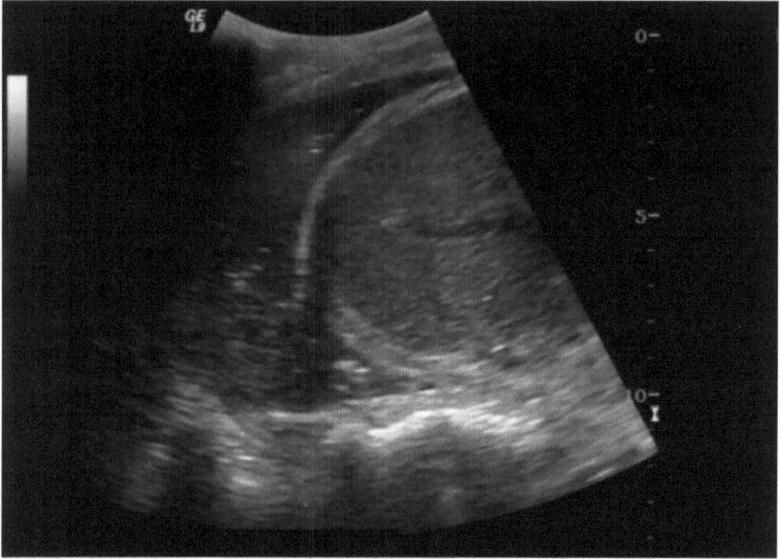

Figure 8.17

There are a number of clues that these echoes are real and represent lung pathology (empyema in this case).

- Clue #1: There is no acoustic mirror present. Recall that acoustic mirrors are always highly reflective large interfaces. When lung air forms a mirror, the reflector is highly echogenic. There is no highly echogenic reflector beyond the diaphragm in this image.

- Clue #2: Real structures (spine, ribs and body wall) are visualized in the dependent part of this image. If the lung contents represented a mirror image artifact of the liver, no real structures would be visualized in the chest.

- Clue #3: The beam is incident on the lung. If the lung was normally inflated with air, it would not be possible to visualize the liver beyond the lung interface.

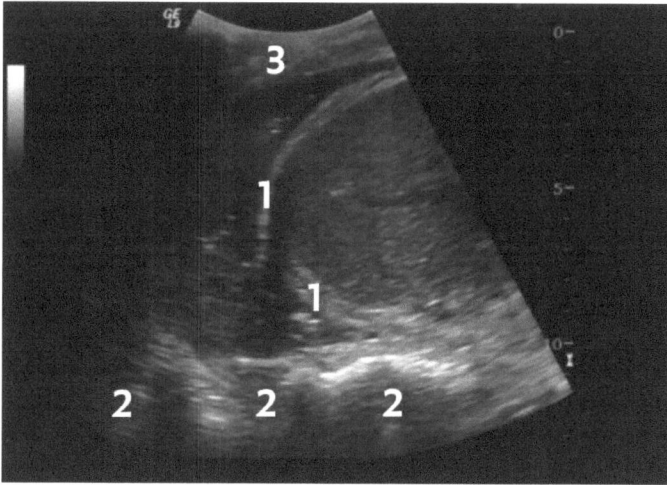

Figure 8.18

Another example

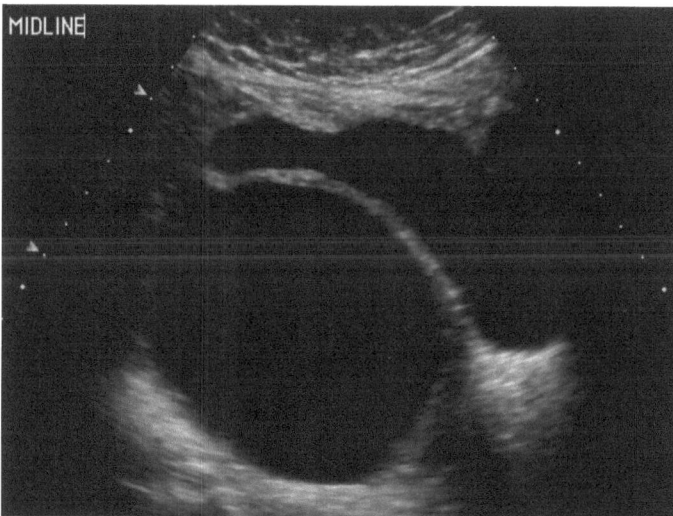

Figure 8.19: Is the cystic mass behind the bladder in this patient a real structure or a mirror-image artifact of the bladder?

The mass is real. It cannot be a mirror image artifact because no mirror is present in the field of view. Specifically, no highly echogenic interfaces are present beyond the bladder wall which could act as acoustic mirrors.

Chapter 9

Reflection Artifact

Reflection or bending of the ultrasound beam can occur at acute angles resulting in apparent displacement of deeper structures. This is a relatively uncommon artifact.

Also known as

Critical angle problem.

Causative mechanisms

Ultrasound beam encounters an interface at a small (acute) angle. Instead of maintaining a straight course, the beam is reflected and changes course.

Which system assumptions have been breached?

The assumption that ultrasound always travels in a straight line.

Typical appearance

Critical angle issues probably occur frequently in ultrasound on small scales, but large scale reflection artifacts are relatively uncommon. When they do occur, they can lead to displacement of distal structures producing apparent breaks in the normal anatomy.

Can this artifact be reduced, eliminated or circumvented?

Changing the angle of approach will eliminate this artifact.

Is this artifact diagnostically useful?

No. The artifact may be confusing to operators because it is uncommon.

Example

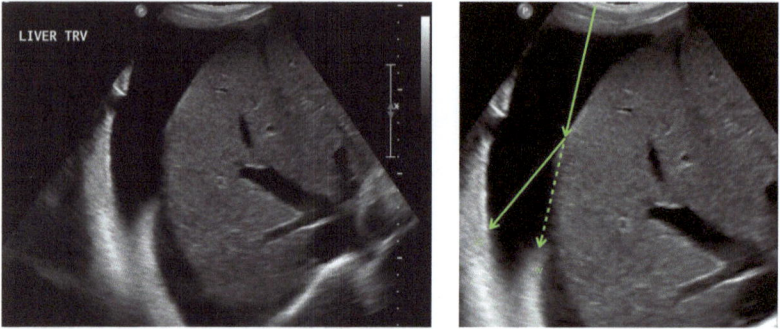

Figure 9.1: The curved liver surface in this patient with ascites causes the ultrasound beam to reflect (solid arrows). Echoes from the lateral abdominal wall (W) then return to the transducer along the same reflected pathway. These echoes are assumed by the system to represent real structures along a straight ultrasound beam represented by the dithered arrow. The abdominal wall is displayed in an incorrect location (w).

Chapter 10

Propagation Speed Artifact

Ultrasound systems assume that the propagation speed of sound is a constant (1540 m/s). Minor variability in the speed of sound, however, exists between tissues of different types. This variability is usually less than 10% and the small differences in propagation speed don't have a significant visual impact on ultrasound images. On rare occasions propagation speed differences can become visible.

Causative mechanisms

A structure of lower or higher propagation speed is present in the field of view adjacent to structures of average propagation speed. Because the system assumes a constant propagation speed (1540m/s) and calculates reflector position on the basis of echo reception time, objects beyond the causative structure are displaced up or down along the lines of sight.

Which system assumptions have been breached?

The assumption that propagation speed of sound is constant.

Typical appearance

Vertical displacement of echoes beyond the causative structure. If the propagation speed of sound in the causative structure is lower than that of surrounding tissues, echoes are displaced downward. Conversely if the propagation speed of sound in the causative structure is greater than that of the surrounding tissues, echoes are displaced upward.

Can this artifact be reduced, eliminated or circumvented?

Propagation speed artifacts cannot be eliminated although a different angle of approach may help. When the scanned tissue is globally of different propagation speed, some manufacturers will permit the operator to make adjustments which assume a different speed of sound.

Is this artifact diagnostically useful?

No. This is a rarely observed artifact which is not useful.

Varicose veins

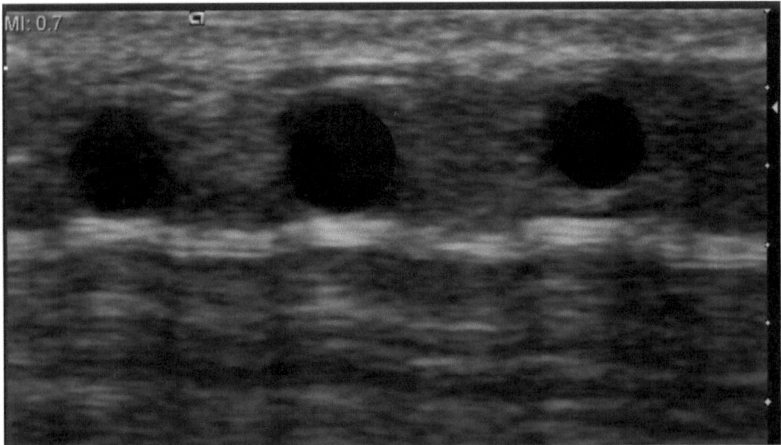

Figure 10.1: Varicose veins provide one example where propagation speed artifacts are commonly observed.

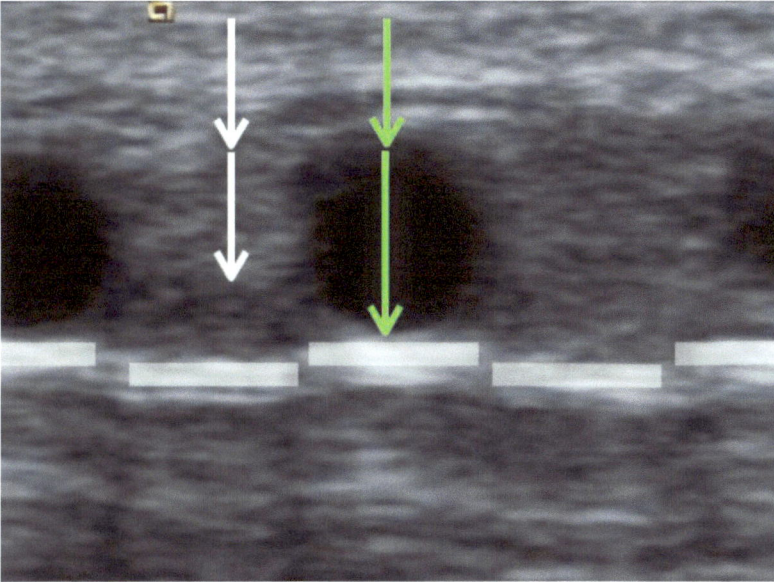

Figure 10.2: Detail showing the causative mechanism of the artifact shown in Figure 10.1.

The propagation speed of sound in blood is fractionally greater than that of the surrounding subcutaneous fat. An acoustic pulse arrives at the deep fascia faster when traveling through the vein (green arrow) than when traveling through subcutaneous fat (white arrows). The echo from the deep fascia is also accelerated on its return trip.

Because pulse-echo time interval is expressed by the system as depth using average propagation speed of sound as a constant, the fascial echo is plotted closer to the transducer.

In this example multiple segments of the varicose vein are crossing the field of view. The deep fascia demonstrates step-like displacement.

Chapter 11

Range Ambiguity

> The range ambiguity artifact is quite a common artifact, but it has complex causation and is therefore often misunderstood by ultrasound operators.

Causative mechanisms

For each scan line on the ultrasound image, the transducer emits a pulse and then waits for the returning echoes before another pulse is emitted. The depth of the FOV determines the required pulse repetition period (PRP) and the corresponding pulse repetition frequency (PRF). Range ambiguity occurs when echoes from a preceding pulse arrive at a time when another pulse-echo sequence is active. The echoes from the preceding and current pulse are co-mingled. Normally, the correct calculation and implementation of PRF prevents echoes from different pulses co-mingling. There are specific circumstances under which echoes do get mixed up. There are two common scenarios where this occurs:

1   The depth of the FOV is relatively shallow but a large low attenuating structure lies beyond the FOV. The initial pulse travels to the bottom of the FOV, echoes are received in the given PRP and then a second pulse is emitted. In the meantime, the initial pulse continues to propagate through a low attenuating structure beyond the FOV. High intensity echoes are generated

beyond the structure and these return at a later time when the second (third, fourth…) pulse is already interrogating the field of view.

2   The system is operating with multiple focal zones. Let's suppose that two focal zones are used. For each scanline, the machine needs to emit a pulse focused at the first focal zone, collect the echoes and then emit a pulse focused at the second focal zone and collect the echoes. The image is stitched together vertically so that the information on top of the display represents echoes received from the first pulse and information on the bottom of the display represents echoes received from the second pulse. Normally, the system waits the entire PRP for each pulse before the next pulse is emitted. However, when multiple focal zones are used, echo information on the bottom of the display belonging to the first pulse will be discarded anyway since it is out of focus. It will be replaced by echo information from the second pulse. In order to achieve better frame rates when multiple focal zones are used, the system does not wait the entire PRP before emitting the next pulse. The system waits only the proportion of the PRP required to gather echoes from the focal region of each pulse. The consequence of this time saving is that the pulse attributable to the first focal zone may continue to propagate and generate echoes after the pulse for the second focal zone has already been emitted. The term 'range ambiguity' pertains to the uncertainty of object location when echoes from this object arrive at some later time.

Which system assumptions have been breached?

The assumption that the arriving echo was generated by the last emitted ultrasound pulse, not any preceding pulses.

Typical appearance

When using curvilinear array transducers, miniature copy (or copies) of the original object can be present within the real object. Alternatively, echogenic band-like image fragments are projected into a large anechoic structure.

Can this artifact be reduced, eliminated or circumvented?

Yes. If the artifact is present and the system is operating with multiple transmit focal zones, switching to a single focal zone will eliminate the artifact. If the artifact is present due to a very low attenuation structure beyond the region of interest (or beyond the FOV), reducing the acoustic output power and gain will reduce the appearance of the artifact.

Some ultrasound systems try to prevent the user from configuring focal zones in a manner that promotes range ambiguity. For example, some systems will not permit the user to set multiple closely spaced focal zones close to the transducer when the image depth is relatively deep.

Unfortunately, some ultrasound systems do not inform the user particularly well as to how many focal zones are being used. Most ultrasound machines show the position of the transmit focal zones as arrowheads on the side of the image.

One manufacturer (Philips) has chosen instead to show a focal "region" which can be increased or decreased by the operator. Effectively what this means is that with a larger focal region the machine will use greater number of focal zones. The operator is not, however, informed how many focal zones are being used. The default system presets are designed so that multiple focal zones are almost always used (not selectively used by operator choice) which means that the system is prone to range ambiguity artifacts as a default. It is up to the operator to avoid the problem by using focal zones positioned in the dependent part of the image or reducing the number of focal zones to one.

Is this artifact diagnostically useful?

No. The artifact is never useful and can lead to bizarre appearances. The operator usually recognizes that an artifact is at play but most operators do not understand the underlying causes of this artifact.

Examples

A large intra-abdominal fluid-filled tumor is shown in Figures 11.1, 11.2 and 11.3. Multiple focal zones are being used as a default machine setting.

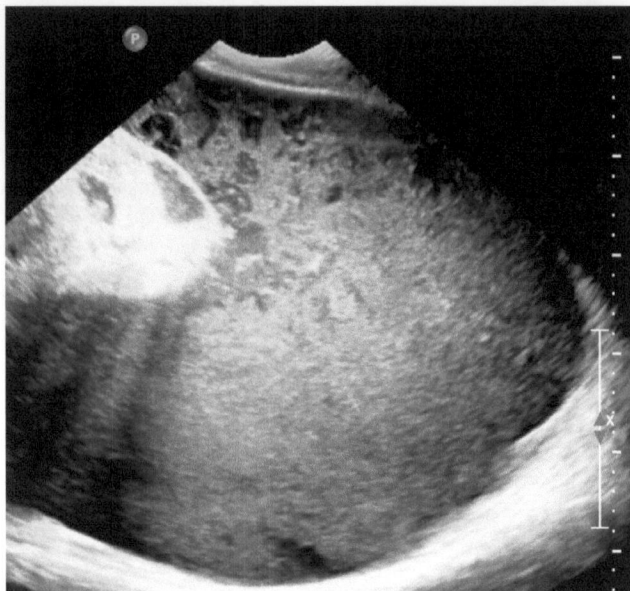

Figure 11.1: When the focal zones are positioned in the dependent part of the image, the mass is correctly represented on the display.

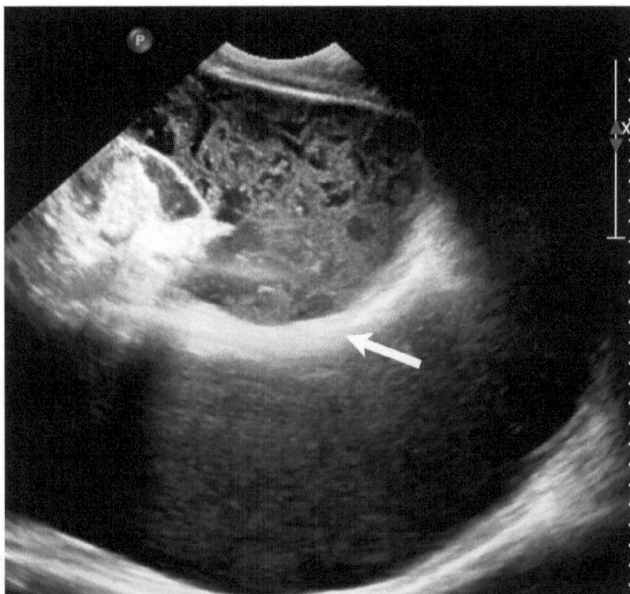

Figure 11.2: If the focal zones are shifted to superficial regions, range ambiguity artifact appears (arrow).

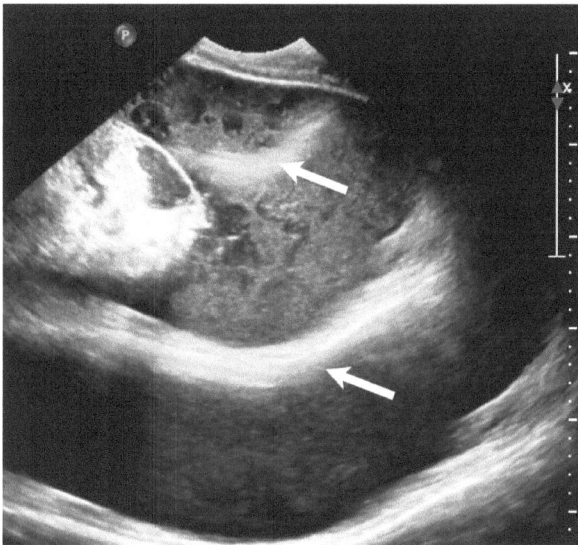

Figure 11.3: Increasing the number of focal zones creates further range ambiguity artifacts (arrows).

Another example of range ambiguity artifact can be seen in this case of abdominal ascites (Figures 11.4 and 11.5).

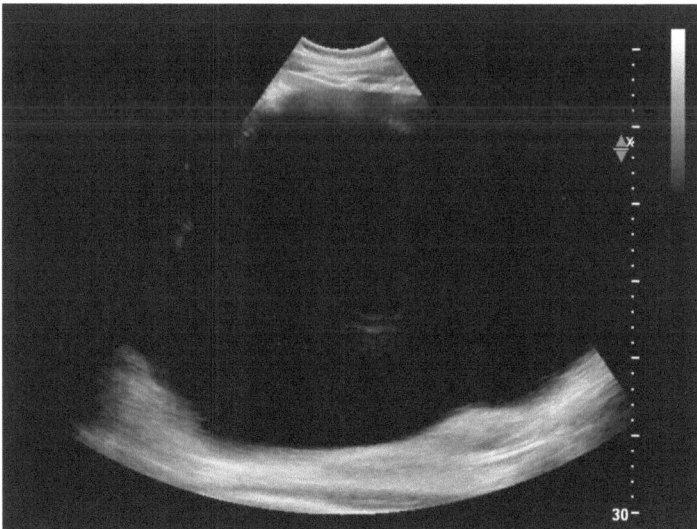

Figure 11.4: The true image is shown here with the abdominal wall at approximately 25cm.

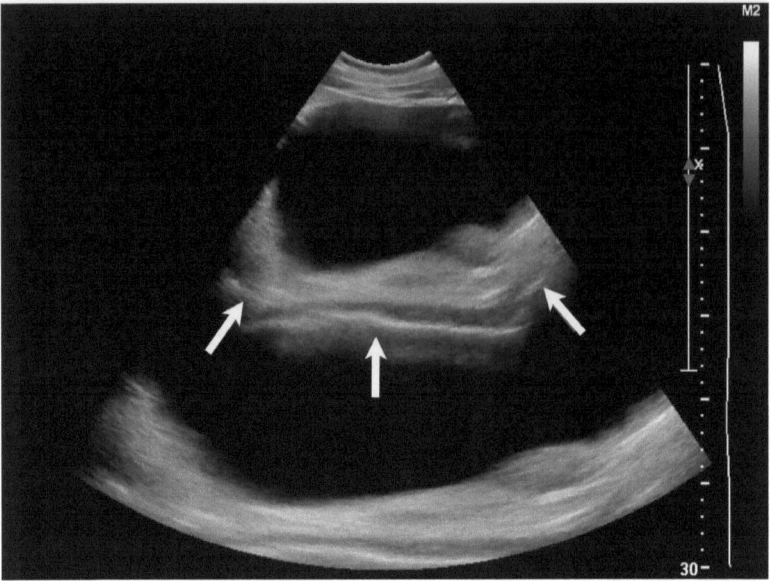

Figure 11.5: When multiple focal zones are used, a miniature copy of the abdominal wall is projected into the true image (arrows) with a second abdominal wall appearing at a depth of approximately 15cm.

A dilemma

This intriguing case (Figures 11.6 to 11.11) caused a real diagnostic dilemma for the sonographer.

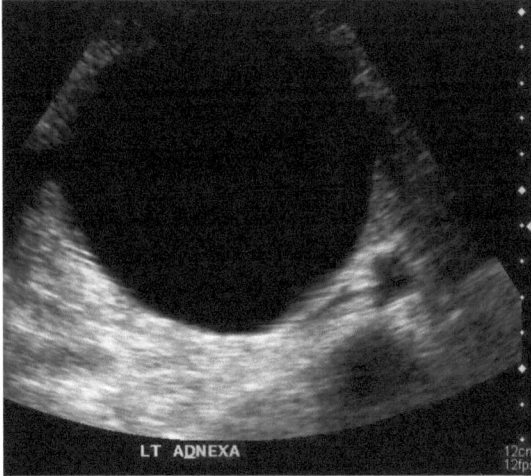

Figure 11.6: Initially a transabdominal scan was performed which demonstrated a simple ovarian cyst.

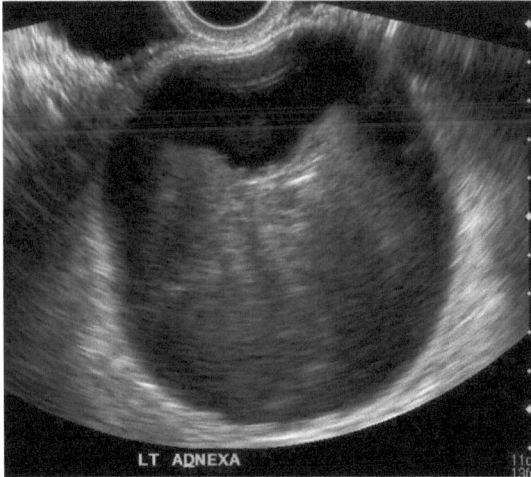

Figure 11.7: The sonographer then performed a transvaginal ultrasound, which revealed that the previously simple anechoic lesion was filled with echoes, effectively qualifying it by IOTA (International Ovarian Tumor Analysis group) criteria as a solid ovarian mass.

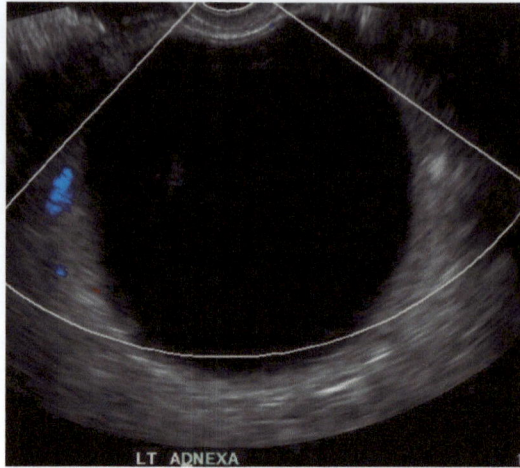

Figure 11.8: To the amazement of the sonographer, when color Doppler was switched on during the transvaginal scan, all internal echoes immediately disappeared and the mass again appeared anechoic.

Believing that the best image quality and best contrast resolution was achieved on greyscale transvaginal imaging, the sonographer made the diagnosis of a complex, predominantly solid ovarian mass. Finally, the sonographer consulted a senior colleague who determined that range ambiguity artifact was at play and confirmed the diagnosis to be a simple cyst. The solution to this case lies in the presence or absence of conditions causing range ambiguity.

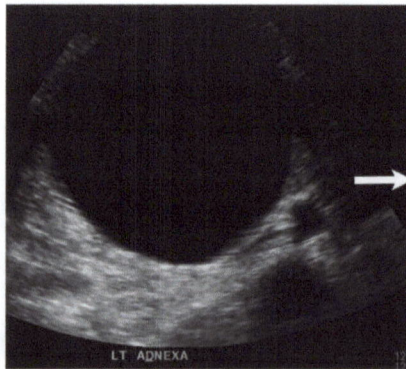

Figure 11.9: The transabdominal scan is performed with a single focal zone (arrow) and range ambiguity does not occur. The image represents the mass accurately as anechoic simple cystic lesion.

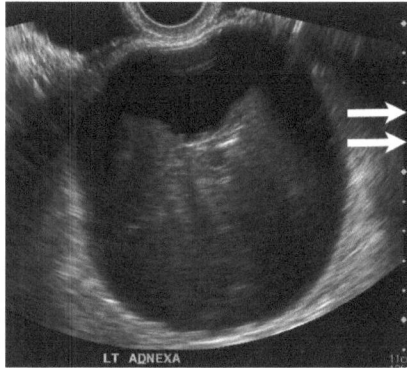

Figure 11.10: When the sonographer switched to the transvaginal transducer, the default system preset for this transducer activated two focal zones (arrows). Because the ovarian mass is relatively large, the sonographer increased the depth of the field of view, but failed to shift the focal zones to the more dependent part of the field of view. This created the perfect conditions for range ambiguity to occur. All the internal echoes are artifactual.

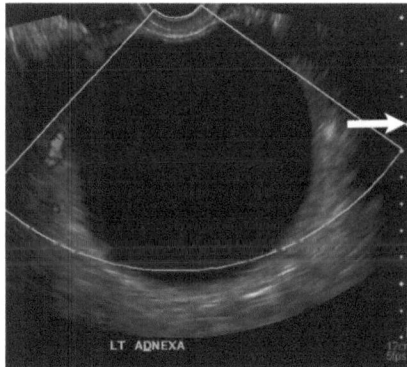

Figure 11.11: When the sonographer switched on color Doppler, the system immediately reverted to using a single focal zone (arrow) because the demands on system resources do not permit multiple focal zones to be used in color Doppler. The range ambiguity artifact disappeared as a consequence.

Chapter 12

Motion Artifact

Image blurring and smearing can sometimes be observed, similar to time-lapse photography. This occurs when the physiologic event is very fast, when the sonographer is moving the transducer too quickly, or when system settings are adjusted in such a way that temporal resolution is poor.

Also known as

Temporal localization artifact, motion blur.

Causative mechanisms

1   Sudden movement of the patient.

2   The observed physiologic event is very fast.

3   The sonographer is moving the transducer too quickly.

4   System settings are adjusted in such a way that temporal resolution is poor.

Which system assumptions have been breached?

The assumption that the rate of image acquisition exceeds

1   the rate of physiologic events and

2   the rate of transducer movement.

Typical appearance

This artifact is very easy to identify as it causes blurring of image along the direction of fast movement.

Common misconceptions

It is a common misconception that temporal resolution is synonymous with frame rate. While it is true that high frame rates are usually associated with high temporal resolution, it is not always the case.

The confusion over frame rate and temporal resolution has not been helped by the complex ways that ultrasound manufacturers calculate effective frame rate. The frame rate displayed on the ultrasound monitor does not usually represent complete frames of information being displayed per second, but rather the ability of the machine to acquire information for a single frame.

Let's consider some examples. In the first scenario the sonographer is scanning the liver with the persistence control (frame averaging) at 0. The sonographer then switches persistence to 5. There is a dramatic loss of temporal resolution following this action because the sonographer is looking at a transparency display of the last 5 frames of information. There is a visible lag in the image refresh rate, but the frame rate displayed by the system will be the same in both instances.

In the second scenario, the sonographer is scanning the liver in conventional (not compounded) mode. The sonographer then switches on spatial compounding at 7 lines of sight per aperture. Again, a dramatic loss of temporal resolution is experienced, but the frame rate displayed by the system will not be substantially different. In conclusion, the frame rate displayed by the ultrasound system is often not a good measure of temporal resolution.

Can this artifact be reduced, eliminated or circumvented?

This artifact can usually be radically reduced or eliminated. If the sonographer is causing motion blur because of fast survey technique, the sonographer can simply slow down. If sudden patient movement causes this artifact, the use of cine-loop will allow the sonographer to rewind the scan in order to record a better quality image.

In circumstances when the sonographer needs to improve temporal resolution due to fast physiologic events (such as cardiac scanning), the options include:

1 Reduce depth of the FOV.
   Trade off: reduction in visible anatomy.

2 Reduce sector width.
   Trade off: reduction in visible anatomy.

3 Reduce the number of focal zones.
   Trade off: less of the FOV in focus.

4 Switch off phase inversion harmonic imaging.
   Trade off: reduction in contrast resolution.

5 Reduce or switch off spatial compounding.
   Trade off: reduction in contrast resolution, more speckle.

6 Reduce or switch off frame averaging.
   Trade off: slight increase in speckle.

7 Lower the line density.
   Trade off: reduction in lateral resolution.

8 Reduce volume density in 3D and 4D imaging.
   Trade off: reduction in slice thickness resolution.

Is this artifact diagnostically useful?

No.

Example

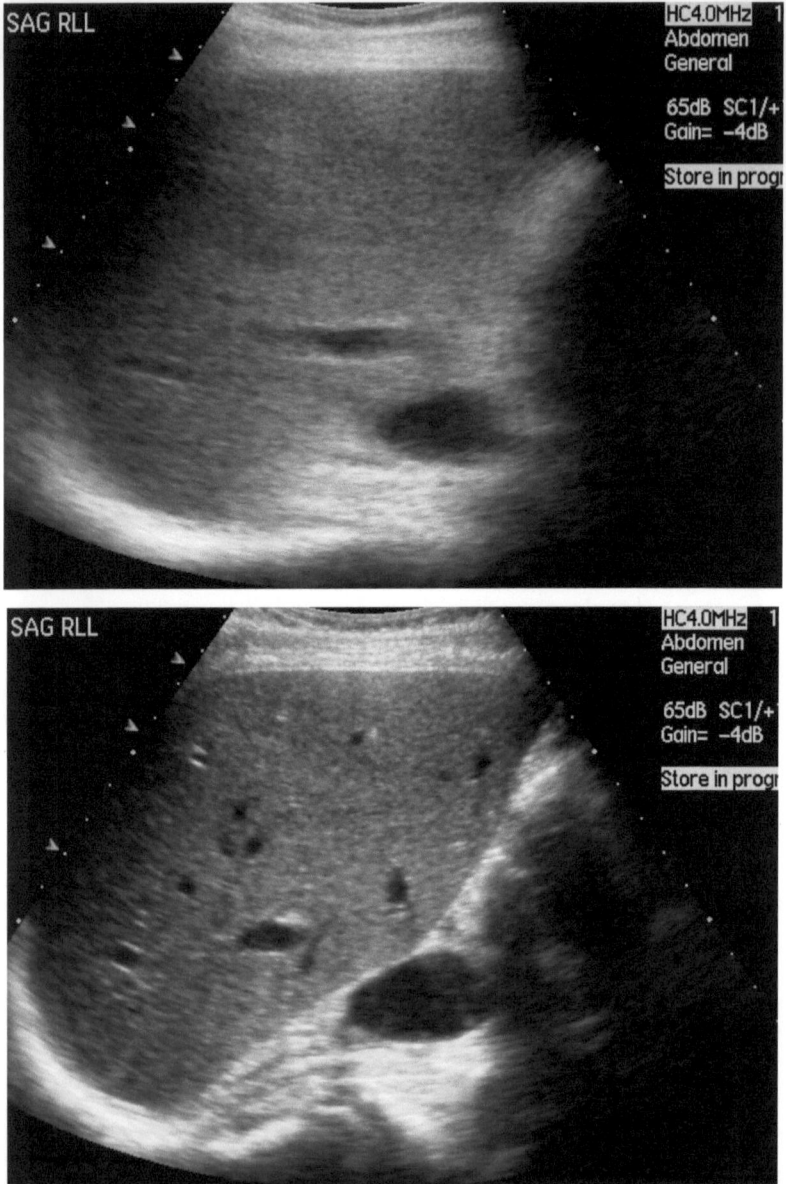

Figure 12.1: Sudden movement of the patient (sneezing) caused a motion artifact during liver imaging (upper image). Rewinding the cine-loop control by a quarter of a second allowed the sonographer to record an identical view without the artifact.

Chapter 13

Acoustic Window and Angle of Approach Effects

Most target organs lie beneath multiple tissue layers that the acoustic pulse must traverse before reaching the region of interest. The acoustic characteristics of these tissues may have a significant impact on the quality of visualization. Homogeneous uniform and low attenuating tissues create the best acoustic windows. Heterogeneous or non-uniform windows may negatively affect visualization. Some of these scenarios have already been discussed including shadowing, dropout, refraction and reverberation. Other scenarios will be presented in this chapter.

Acoustic window

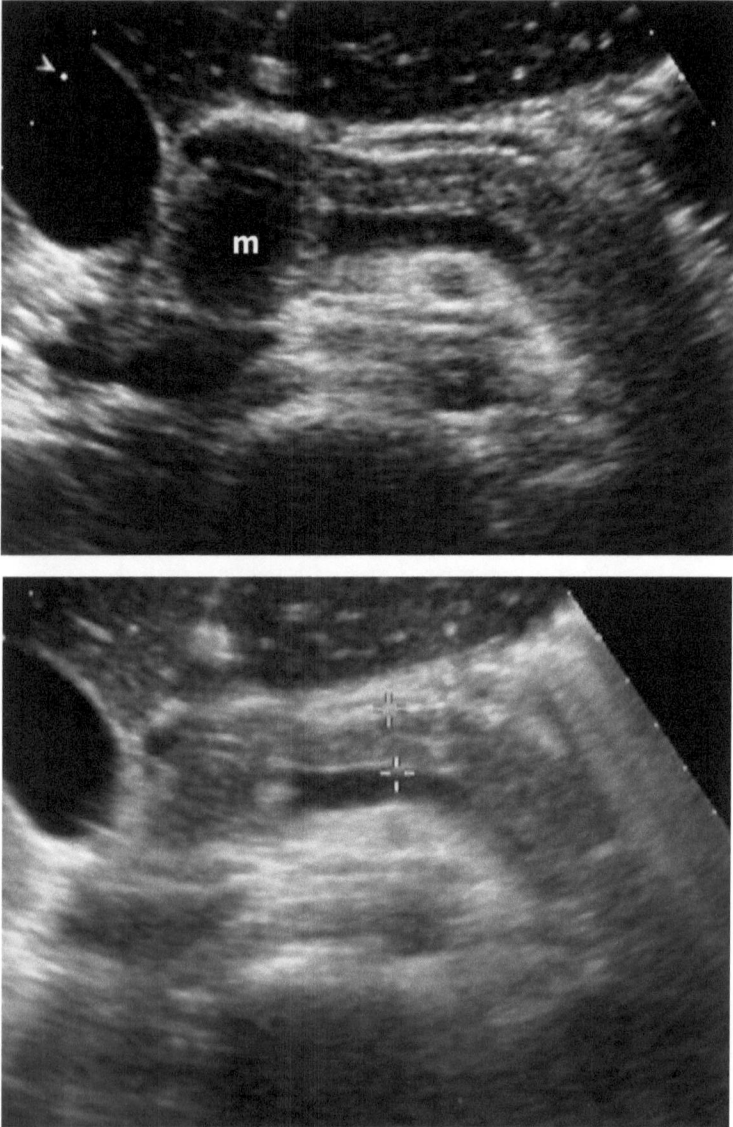

Figure 13.1: (Top) The sonographer used a non-uniform window (falciform ligament and ligamentum teres) to visualize the head of the pancreas. The appearance is highly worrying and suggests the presence of a pancreatic head mass (m). (Bottom) Review of the same area from a different angle revealed a normal pancreatic head.

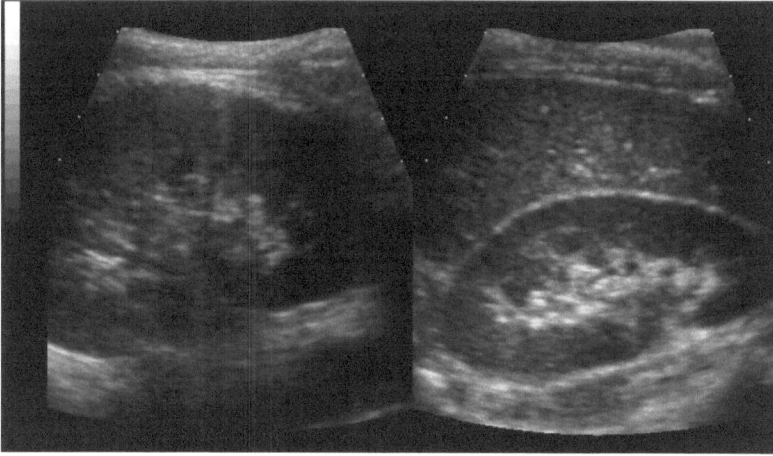

Figure 13.2: The same right kidney was scanned using two different acoustic windows: lateral abdominal wall (left frame) and transhepatic (right frame). The liver provides a more uniform acoustic window resulting in a more homogeneous image with fewer artifacts and better contrast resolution.

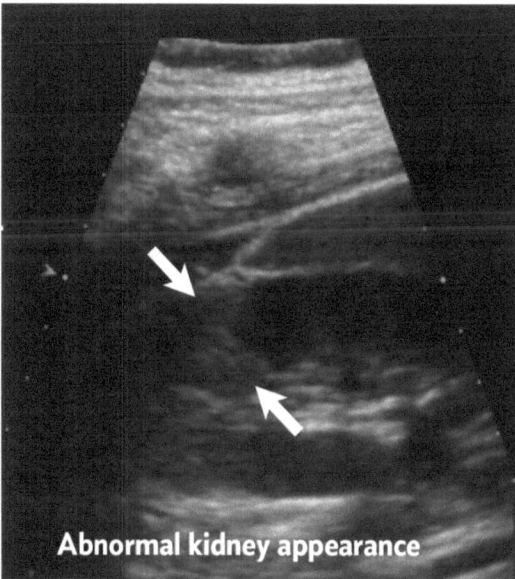

Figure 13.3: A textural abnormality with a vague mass appearance (arrows) was identified in this kidney. Figure 13.4 shows a surveillance scan performed on this kidney a few months later.

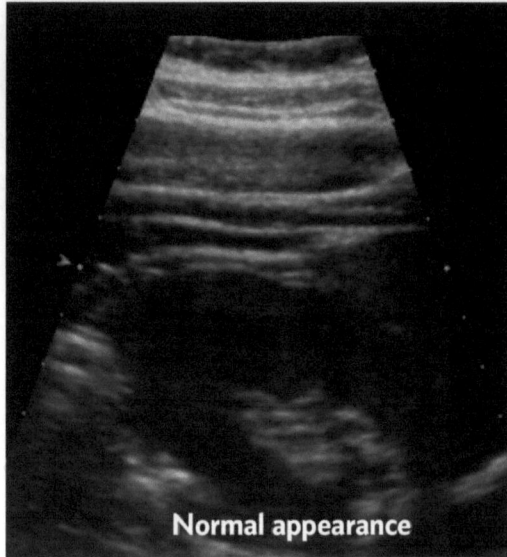

Figure 13.4: This surveillance scan performed a few months later shows that the apparent textural abnormality in the kidney shown in Figure 13.3 is related to non-uniformity of the acoustic window. The appearance disappears if the kidney is scanned through uniform tissues.

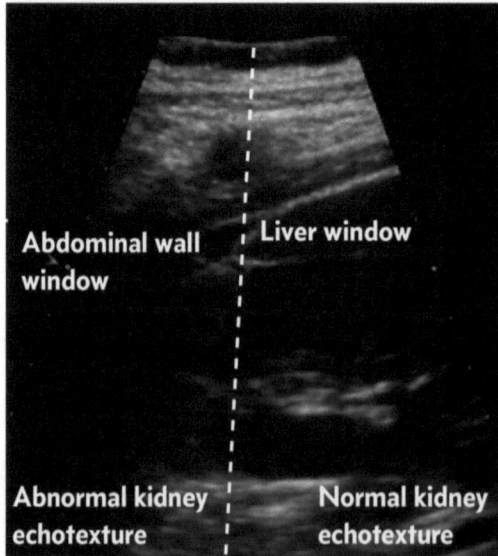

Figure 13.5: Further detail of the kidney image shown in Figure 13.3.

The conspicuity of lesions is heavily dependent on the characteristics of the acoustic window.

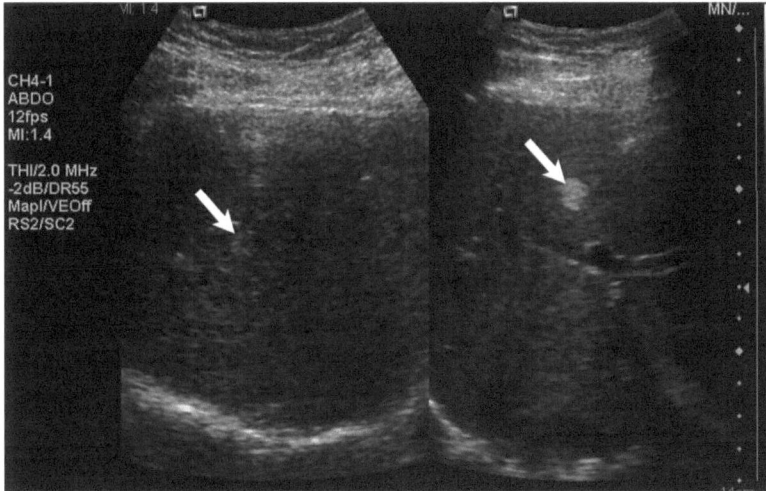

Figure 13.6: In these images, the same liver mass (hemangioma) is scanned using two different approaches. The mass is barely detectable in the left frame whereas it is very obvious in the right frame.

Because the effect of the acoustic window on visualization of structures is difficult to predict, it is important to scan each organ from a variety of approaches and acoustic windows.

For example, it is good practice to always survey the liver in supine subcostal, supine intercostal, decubitus subcostal and decubitus intercostal windows.

Transabdominal and transvaginal images of the same multilocular cystic ovarian tumor are shown below. Even though the mass is well visualized transabdominally, the transvaginal scan demonstrates much better spatial and contrast resolution and provides further important diagnostic clues.

These include: improved septal characterization, fluid compartments with different echogenicity fluid, small septal solid components.

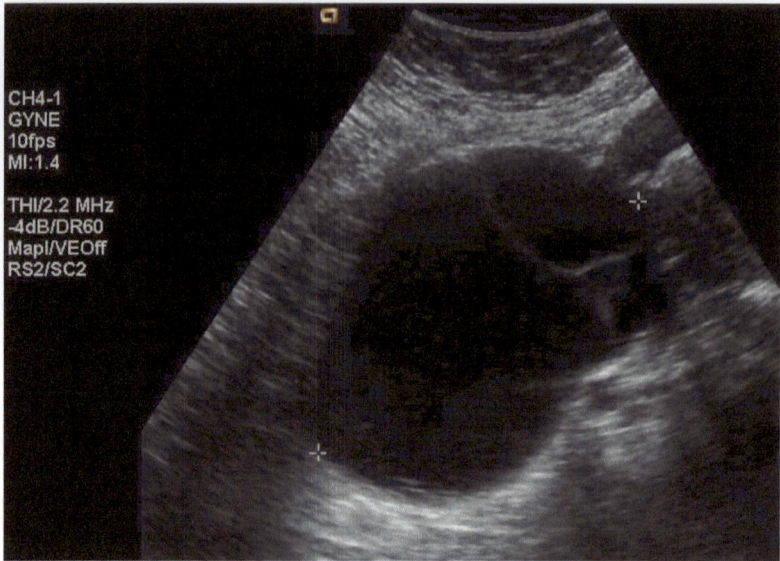

Figure 13.7: Transabdominal image of a multilocular cystic ovarian tumor.

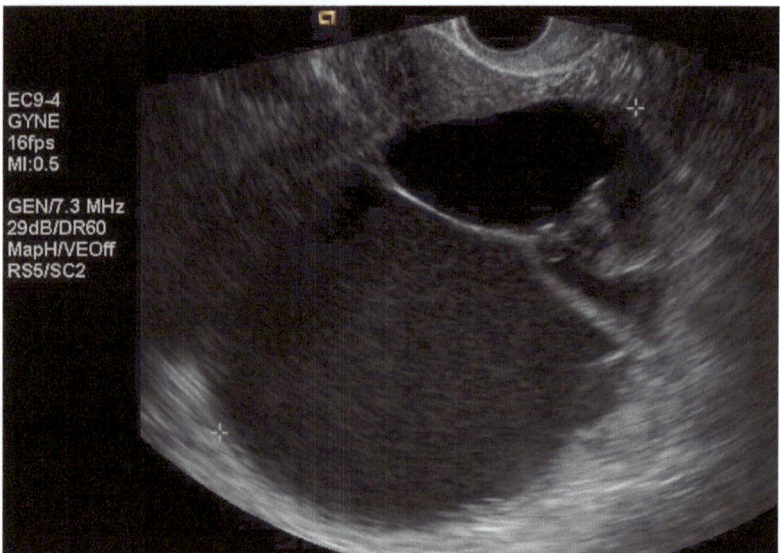

Figure 13.8: Transvaginal image of the tumor shown in Figure 13.7.

Angle of Approach

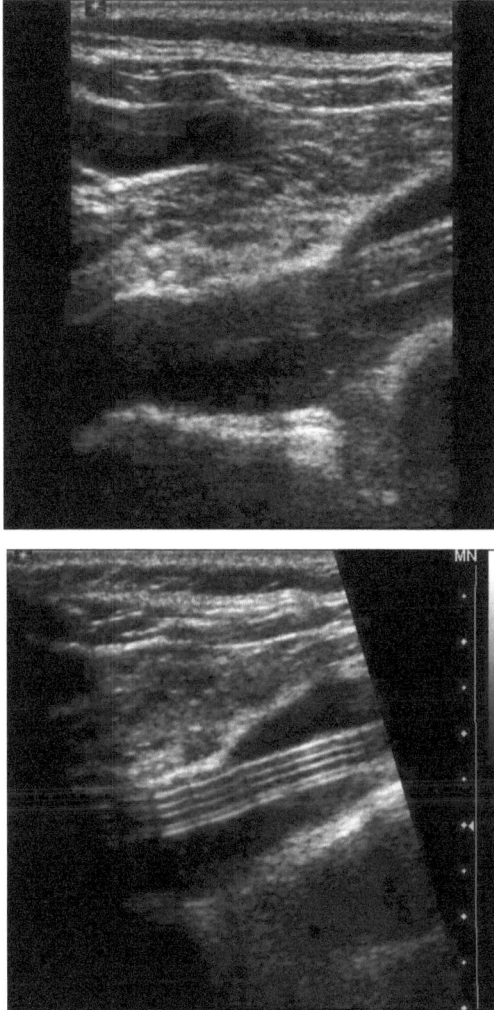

Figure 13.9: A plastic catheter is resting within the left brachiocephalic vein from the supraclavicular window. Visualization of the catheter is poor in the upper image because the beam and catheter are not at normal incidence. Manual angling of the transducer is difficult in this region. The sonographer therefore utilized electronic beam steering to achieve normal incidence (lower image). Visualization of the catheter is dramatically improved because 1) the walls of the catheter are interrogated along the beam axis taking advantage of axial resolution and 2) the reflection coefficient is highest at normal incidence.

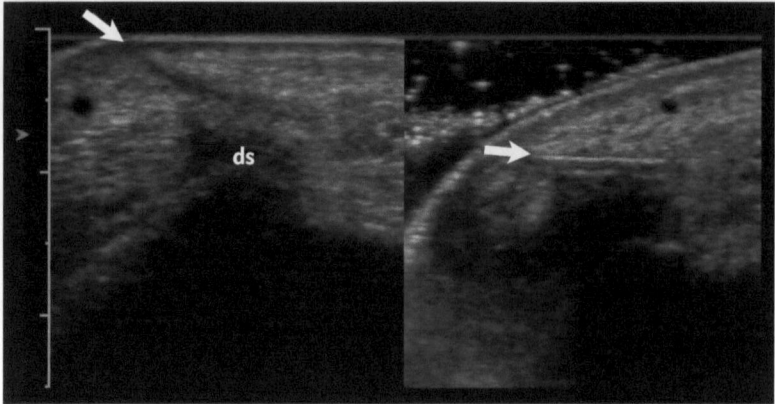

Figure 13.10: This patient presented for ultrasound localization of a suspected foreign body (wooden splinter) in the foot. Initial survey of the region of interest (left image) only revealed the track of soft tissue injury (arrow) with some dirty shadowing (ds). Application of a gel layer to create an acoustic standoff allowed sufficient angulation of the transducer to achieve a 90° approach to the soft tissue track revealing the foreign body within (right image, arrow).

Scanning for foreign bodies is highly angle sensitive. Careful angulation or use of beam steering is often required to visualize foreign bodies. The same applies to a wide variety of iatrogenic devices such as needles, catheters, intravascular lines, wires, sheaths, surgical mesh, synthetic graft material, intrauterine and subcutaneous contraceptive devices and similar objects.

An unfavorable angle of approach created a real diagnostic dilemma in a third trimester gestation presenting for routine assessment of fetal growth (see Figures 13.11, 13.12 and 13.13).

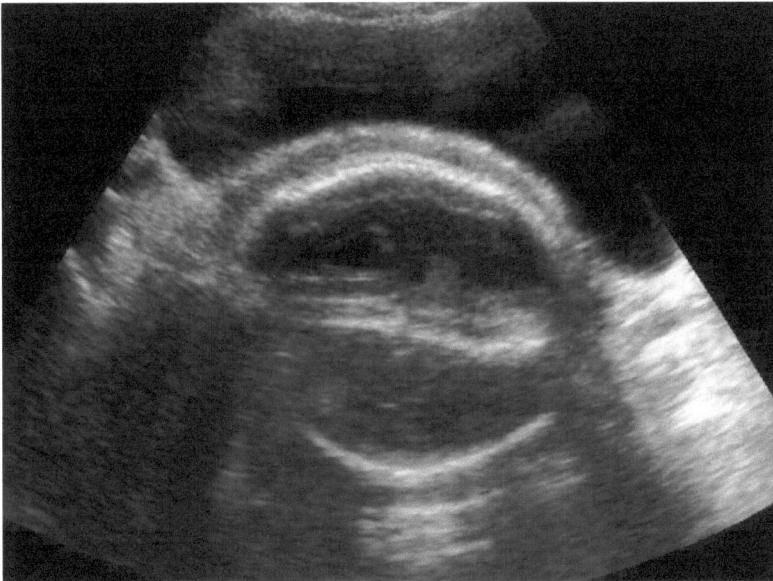

Figure 13.11: The initial transabdominal scan revealed an unusual intracranial appearance.

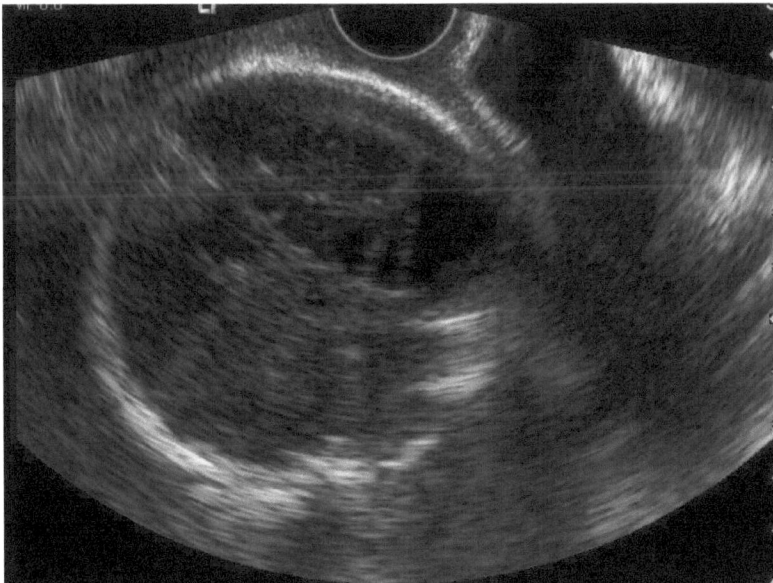

Figure 13.12: The sonographer then switched to transvaginal imaging, which was unhelpful.

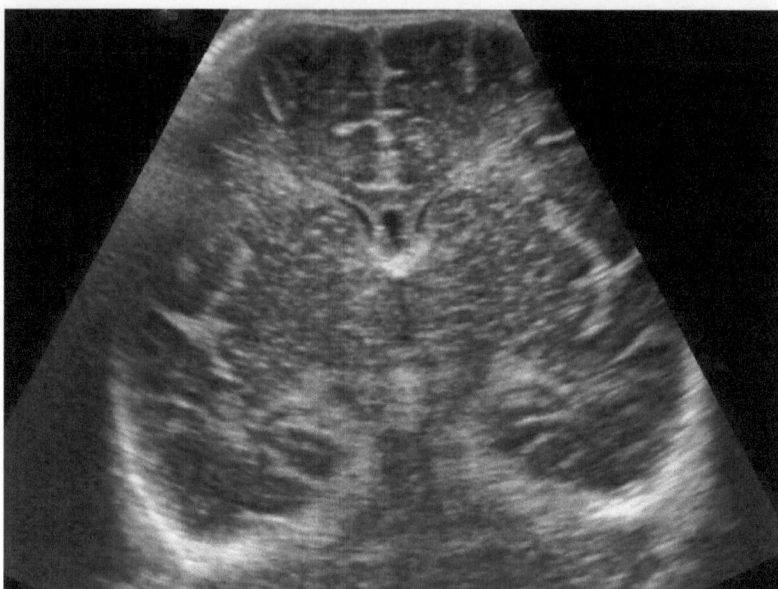

Figure 13.13: Concerned that these appearances may represent true intracranial abnormality, the sonographer organized a postnatal ultrasound. This revealed a perfectly normal brain in this healthy newborn. The cause of the unusual antenatal appearance almost certainly stems from unfavorable fetal lie and the inability of the sonographer to achieve a good angle of approach transabdominally or transvaginally.

Chapter 14

System Artifacts and Malfunctions

The digital nature of modern ultrasound machines makes these systems highly reliable. If a major component of the system malfunctions, the effect is usually a failure of the system to operate altogether. Minor system malfunctions and errors in image processing can produce a wide range of image defects.

Electrical interference

Ultrasound transducers and electronic circuit boards contain highly sensitive components. Strong electrical interference from other nearby electrical devices can, on rare occasion, produce visible interference patterns, as shown below.

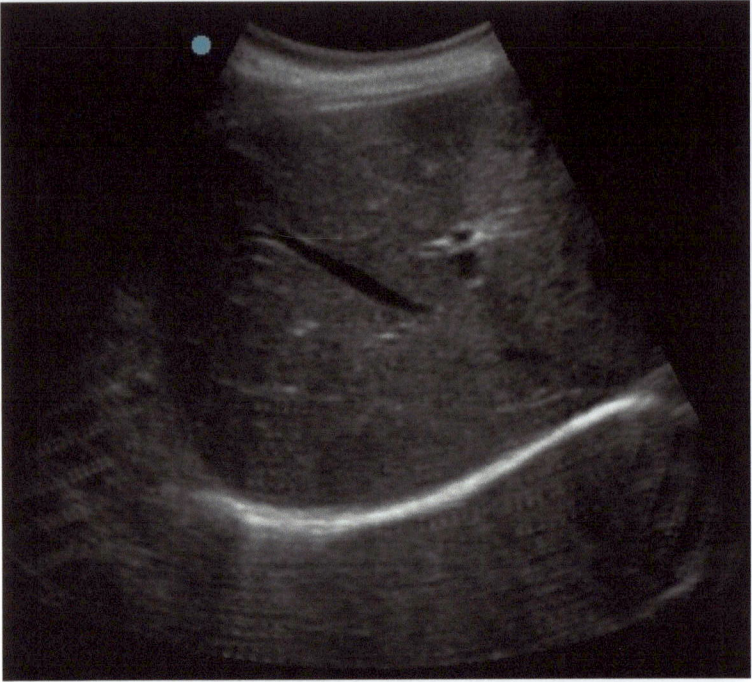

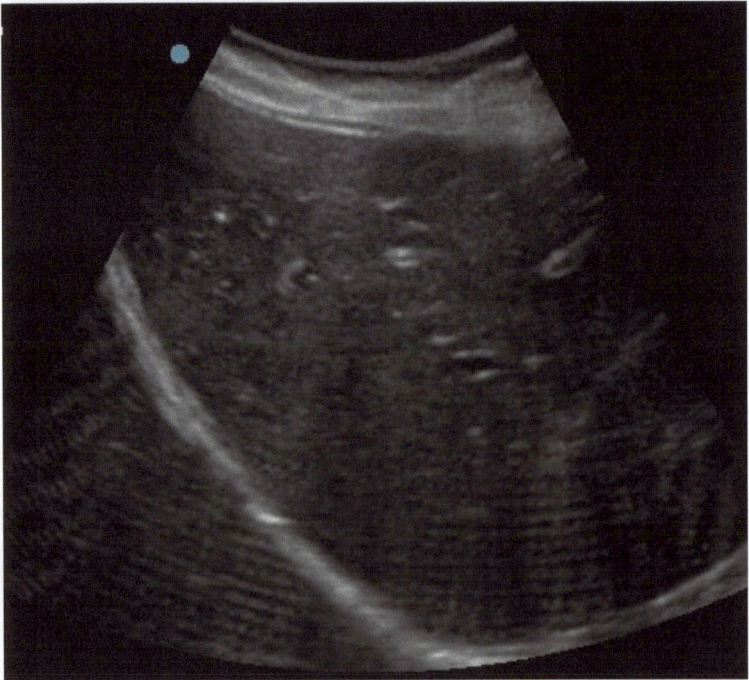

Faulty elements

Faulty transducer elements, poor electrical connections at the transducer port or faulty electronics affecting the performance of individual channels can produce a range of image defects. In the past, missing vertical scan lines were the most evident defects. With the advent of spatial image compounding as a default scanning mode, however, missing scan lines are often masked by active scan lines from adjacent apertures and are much less obvious.

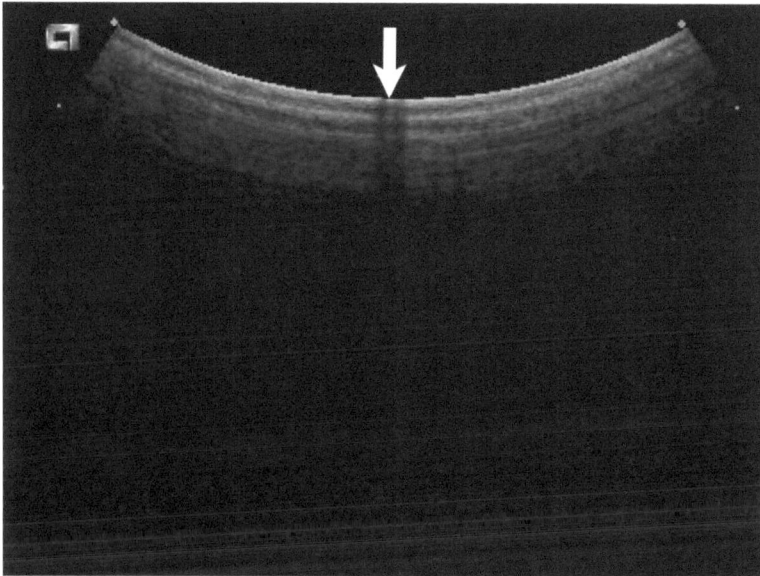

Figure 14.1: A simple uniformity test that best reveals the presence of faulty elements involves applying a small amount of acoustic gel to the surface of the transducer and then running a finger back and forth along the scan head. Faulty elements leave a visible gap.

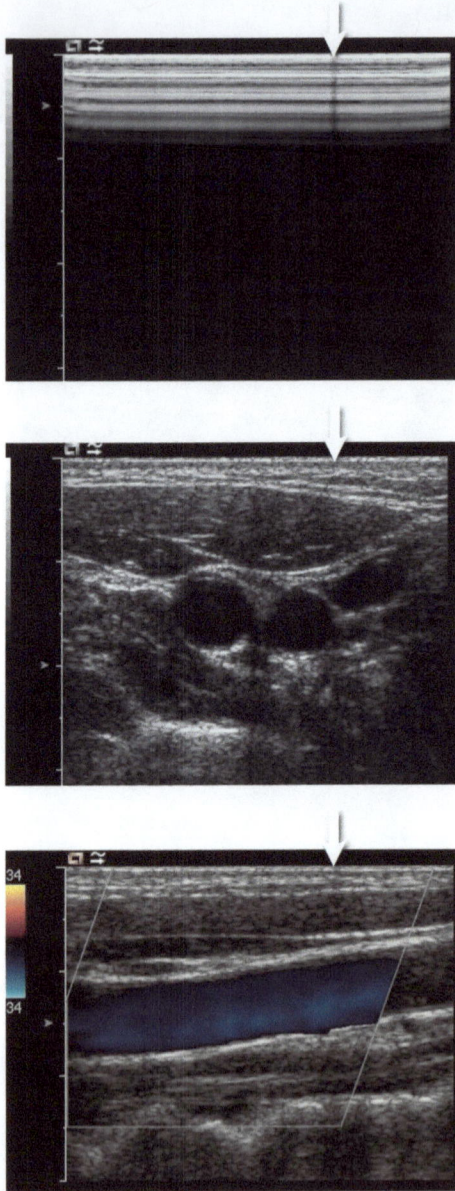

Figure 14.2: A uniformity test performed on this transducer revealed a faulty element (top image), however, the defect is not noticeable at all in the clinical 2D (middle) and color Doppler (bottom) images. This is because a single element makes only a modest contribution to beam formation.

Stitching artifact

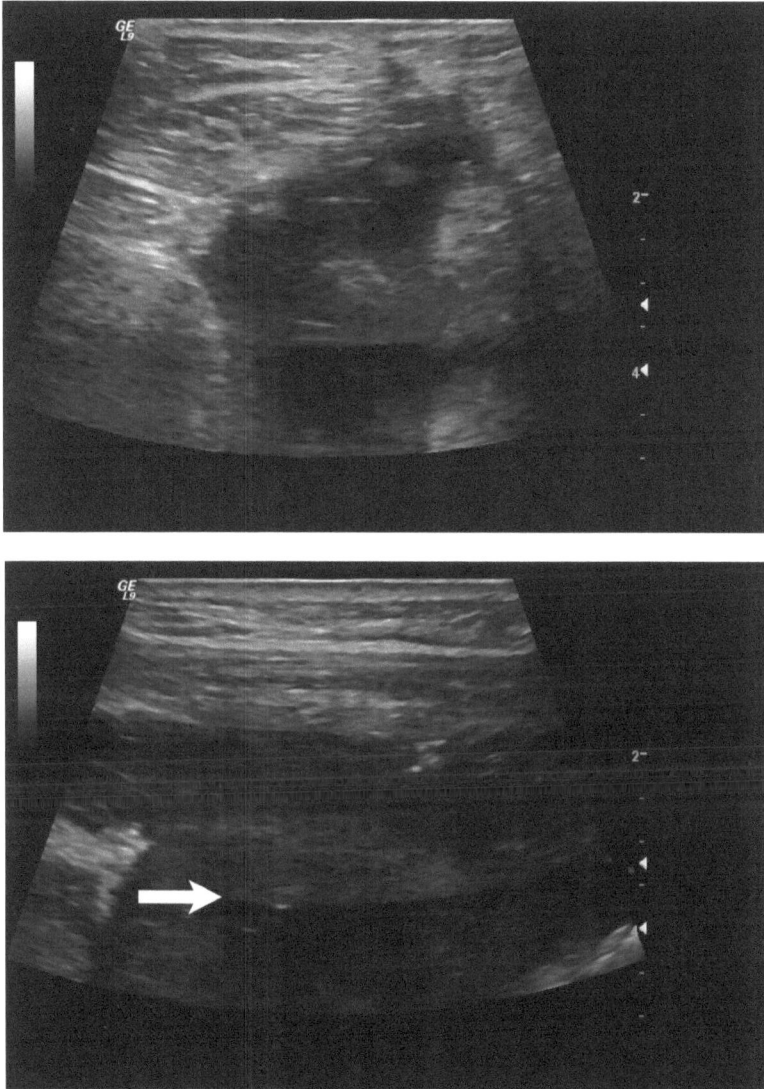

Figure 14.3: Images obtained in multifocal imaging mode are horizontally stitched from echo information belonging to different beams focused at different levels in the image. When automatic gain compensation algorithms fail to accurately amplify echoes, there may be an obvious horizontal break in the image, known as a stitching artifact (arrow).

Panoramic imaging artifacts spatial correlation algorithm problems

The spatial correlation algorithm that tracks image movement in panoramic imaging may fail to correctly construct an image, resulting in discontinuity, steps, empty wedges and other unsightly defects. This can happen for a number of reasons:

1   The sonographer did not move the transducer smoothly and consistently.

2   There was a loss of contact between the transducer and the patient (for example due to a lack of gel or a gas bubble in gel).

3   The soft tissue under the transducer was being compressed as the transducer was swept over the area of interest. This problem occurs particularly when curvilinear transducers are used. Tissue compression is more pronounced directly under the central part of the scan head and less pronounced at the edges. This leads to tissue distortion as the transducer is swept along the region of interest. The tissue distortion creates small amounts of vertical movement in the soft tissue and this is misinterpreted as transducer movement, not tissue movement. The most common distortion resulting from this process is that of concave appearance of a body surface which is otherwise flat or convex.

4   Bowel gas was present in the deeper parts of the FOV. Bowel gas causes a range of artifacts (total shadowing, dirty shadowing, ringdown). Additionally, bowel gas tends to be mobile with peristalsis. These factors contribute to difficulty in accurately tracking the transducer position.

Panoramic spatial-correlation failure

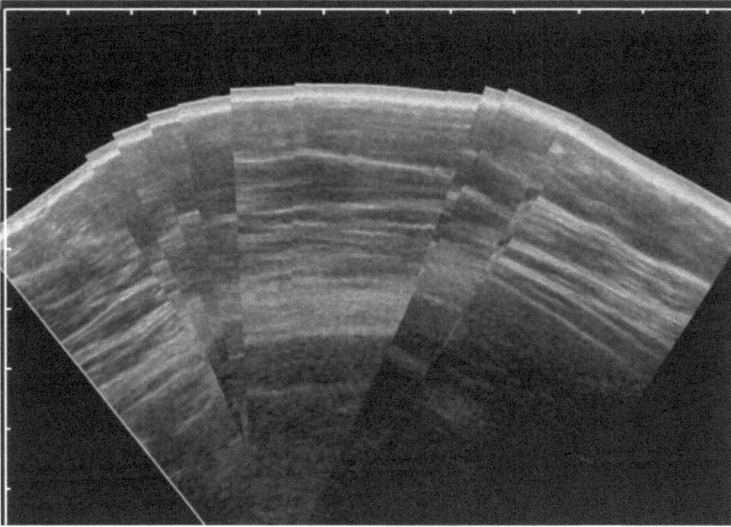

Figure 14.4: This panoramic image acquisition of the abdominal wall demonstrates a failure of the image tracking algorithm due to the presence of bowel gas within the field of view.

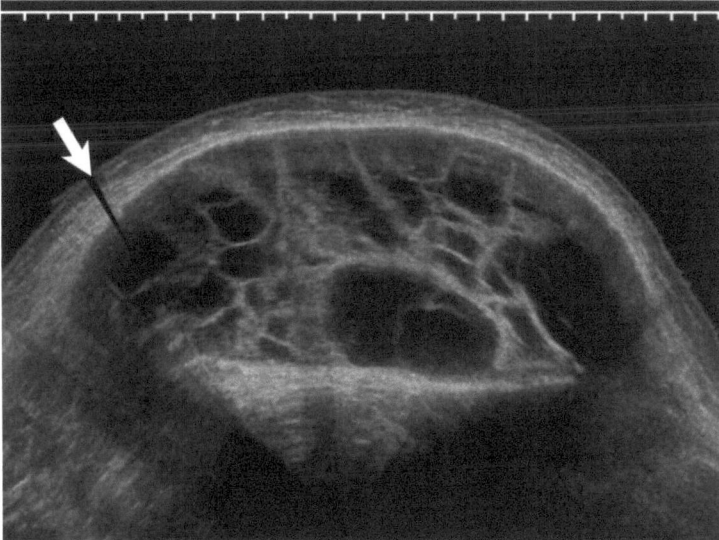

Figure 14.5: A wedge-shaped image defect is evident in this otherwise good-quality panoramic image of a large abdominal wall seroma.

Panoramic tissue distortion problem

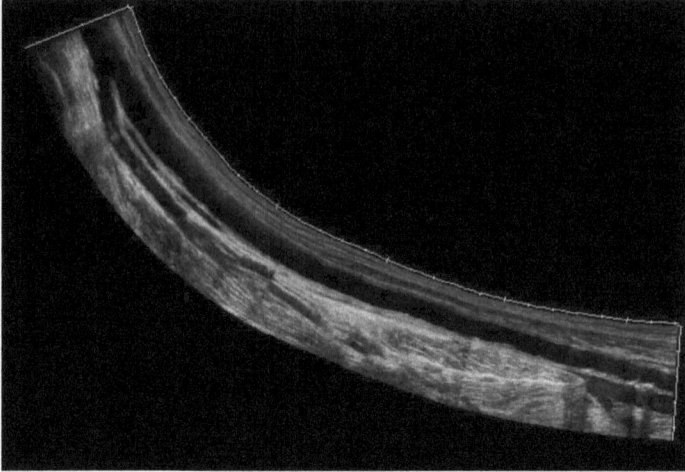

Figure 14.6: This panoramic image of the femoral arterial tree from the common femoral artery (CFA), profunda femoris artery (PFA) and femoral artery (FA) is well reconstructed apart from the curvature. The lower extremity should have a slightly convex, not concave contour. This type of distortion is often caused by tissue compression as the transducer is passed over the tissue which introduces some unexpected horizontal displacement of echoes and confuses the image tracking algorithm.

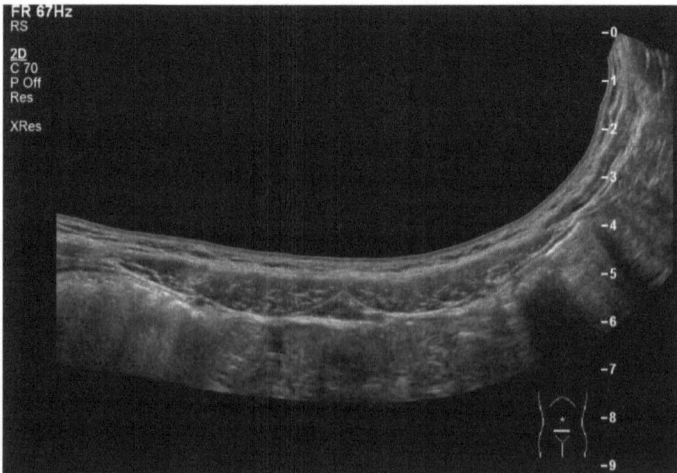

Figure 14.7: Compression during panoramic sweep produces tissue distortion effects which result in concave appearance of the abdominal wall.

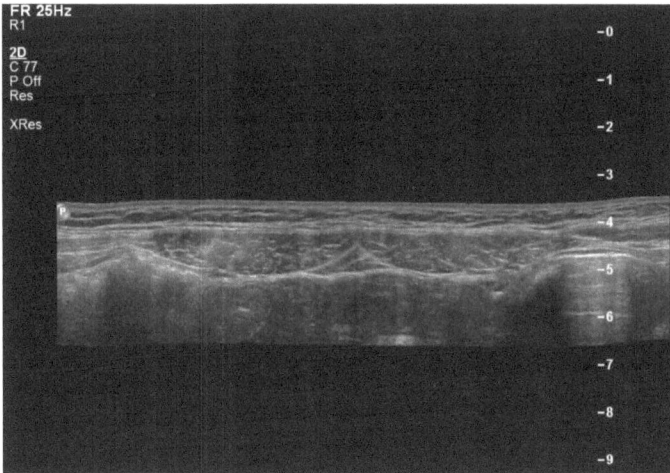

Figure 14.8: Careful panoramic acquisition in the same patient as Figure 14.7 without compression yields an accurate result.

Image composition artifacts

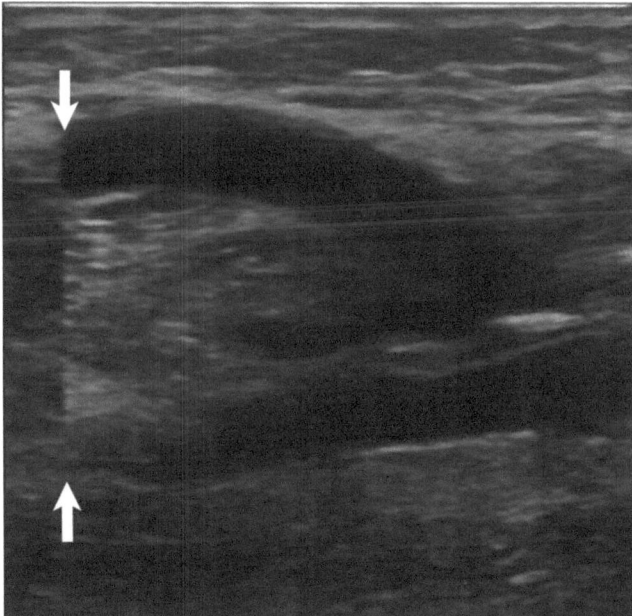

Figure 14.9: Malfunction of the scan converter in this image leads to a vertical defect. The precise cause of the defect is unknown.

Major system malfunctions

Major system malfunctions that produce garbled images without causing software errors and alerting the operator are becoming relatively rare. Most of the time, these events are very easy to recognize.

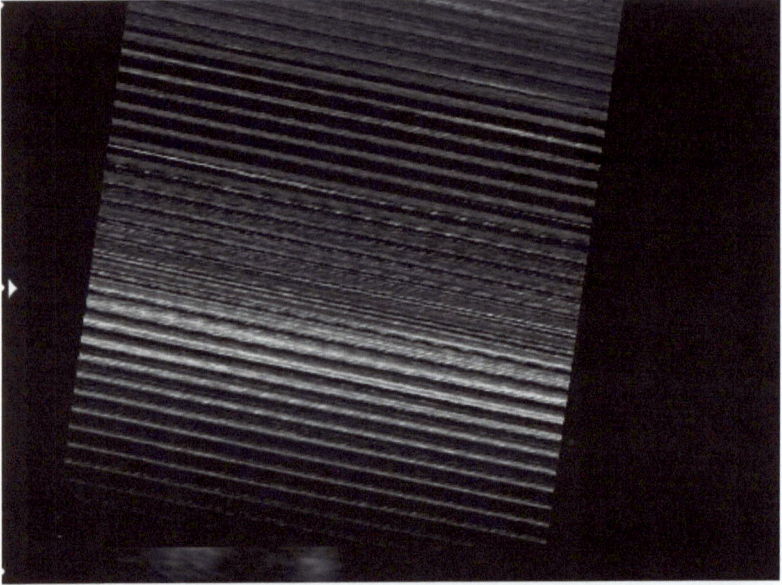

Image courtesy Stephen Bird, Adelaide

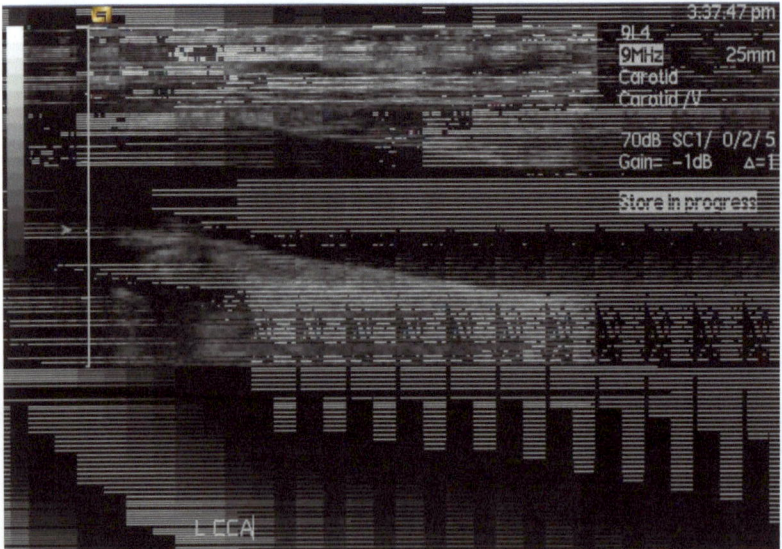

Chapter 15

Artifact Avoidance Strategies

With all the vast range of greyscale artifacts, where does the sonographer even begin in the quest for artifact avoidance? This final chapter includes some basic strategies.

Ultrasound is an interactive imaging modality. The quality of the examination is influenced by the expertise of the operator, their scanning technique, system settings and the quality of the system components. There is no magic strategy which will always reduce artifacts and improve image quality, however, there are several general rules which form a foundation of good ultrasound scanning:

1. **Ultrasound machine**: modern high-end ultrasound scanners always outperform low-end rivals and older machines. If you have a choice of systems to use, select a higher quality machine.

2. **Transducer frequency**: use the highest frequency transducer possible as long as penetration is adequate. Higher frequency transducers bring many benefits: high axial, lateral, slice thickness and contrast resolution, more directional beams with less divergence and usually higher element density. Many systems also offer frequency compounding options which are often advantageous.

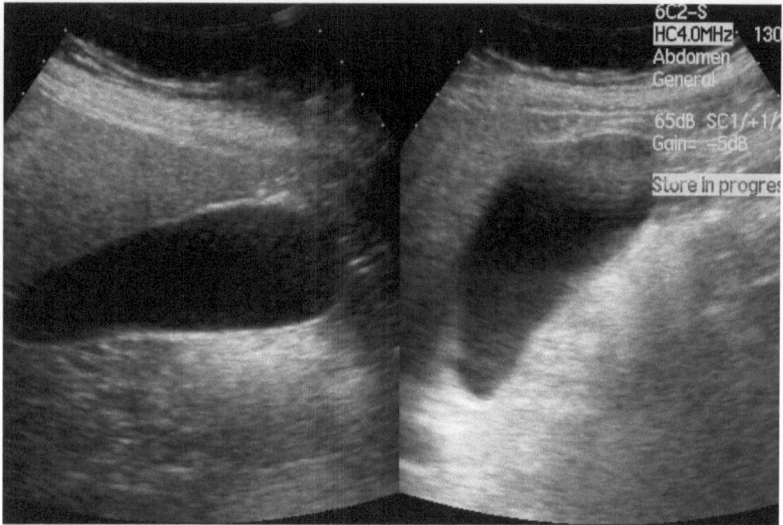

Figure 15.1: The same gallbladder scanned from two different approaches using the same transducer and identical system settings yields dramatically different image quality. The image in the left frame is clear and conclusive. The image on the right is riddled with artifacts and is non-diagnostic.

3   **Acoustic window**: find a homogeneous uniform acoustic window. Most body structures can be scanned from a variety of approaches. Dramatic improvements in image quality can be achieved by using favorable windows.

4   **Angle of approach**: tubular and striated structures (vessels, ducts, muscles, tendons, ligaments, foreign bodies, plastic lines, stents) as well as organ surfaces and tissue boundaries produce the best results when scanned at normal incidence (90° approach). Unfortunately a perpendicular approach promotes the formation of the reverberation artifact.

5   **Focusing**: focusing reduces beam dimensions and improves lateral resolution. Always set the focal position at the level of the region of interest. Multiple focal zones can be used, but at the expense of temporal resolution.

6   **Gain and TGC**: under most clinical imaging circumstances a slight reduction in gain will often improve contrast resolution.

7   **Tissue harmonic imaging**: harmonic imaging improves contrast resolution and reduces the majority of artifacts. The drawback is usually some tradeoff in axial resolution, penetration and temporal resolution.

8   **Spatial image compounding**: spatial image compounding reduces speckle and the majority of artifacts. It improves contrast resolution, border definition and general lesion conspicuity. The tradeoff is lower temporal resolution as well as reduction in some diagnostically useful imaging artifacts such as distal acoustic shadowing.

9   **High definition zoom**: also known as 'write' or 'pre-processing' zoom can substantially improve image quality, particularly lateral and temporal resolution. Enlargement of the region of interest is also helpful in assessing small structures.

10 **Making wise use of other controls**: a wide range of other system controls are at the disposal of the operator including: dynamic range, edge enhancement, greyscale maps, line density, persistence, reject level and others. While an adjustment of any one of these controls may bring a relatively modest benefit, simultaneous adjustments of multiple controls can have additive effect, leading to a dramatic improvement in the diagnostic quality of the image.

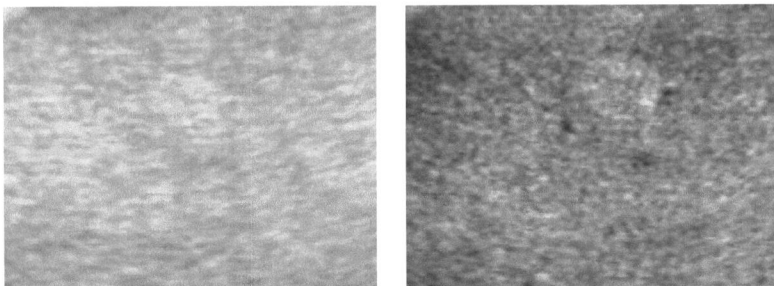

Figure 15.2: In this example, a small isoechoic hemangioma was difficult to appreciate in the initial images (left). Adjustments in multiple system parameters were needed to reveal its presence (right image).

Ultimately, the skill and expertise of the operator has the greatest effect on the overall quality of the diagnostic ultrasound scan.

As with other forms of professional endeavor, a great degree of experience is required to successfully perform ultrasound scans, avoid artifacts and interpret ultrasound images. What separates a good ultrasound practitioner from an expert is probably somewhere in the vicinity of 10,000 hours (Malcolm Gladwell, 2008).

Index

* 9 7 8 0 9 8 7 2 9 2 1 6 2 *